改訂版 クインテッセンス歯科英会話シリーズ

英語で患者と話そう！

PART 1

ENGLISH CONVERSATION FOR DENTIST-PATIENT COMMUNICATION

Thomas R. Ward 著

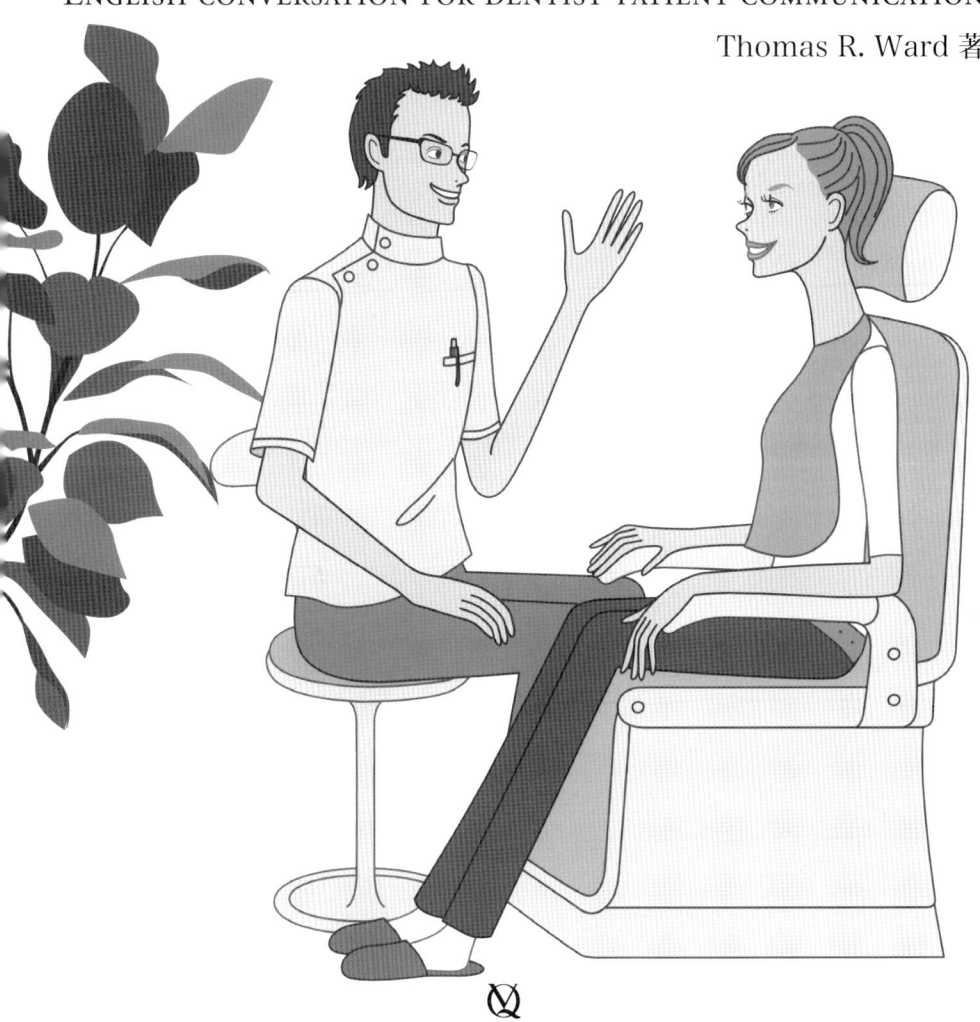

クインテッセンス出版株式会社　2007

Tokyo, Berlin, Chicago, London, Paris, Barcelona, Istanbul, Milano, São Paulo, Moscow, Prague, Warsaw, New Delhi, Beijing, and Bukarest

まえがき

　本書は、歯科医やスタッフが外国人患者とコミュニケーションを持つ際に手助けになるように書かれたものである。現在、日本には200万人以上の外国人が住んでいる。さらに、毎年、700万人を越える人々が、日本を訪れている。日本の国際化を示す証拠となるものだが、この数はますます増えていくようである。この外国人は、開発途上国からの留学生、教師、ビジネスマン、外交官など、さまざまな職業や国籍の人々である。

　われわれ日本で開業している歯科医師とこうした外国人患者とのコミュニケーションを図るうえでは、いろいろな問題が起こりかねない。一般的にいって外国人は、日本人に比べて自分の受ける治療の説明を求めることが多いようである。また、国や職業の違いのため、患者が歯科治療に何を期待しているか、はっきりとつかみにくいこともある。本書では、歯科医とスタッフが、日常の診療で、外国人患者と話すとき役立つような基本的会話を集めてみた。英会話に興味をお持ちの歯科関係者および日常臨床で英語を使う機会のある方々に役立つことを願って企画した。

　なお、本書の出版に際しては、クインテッセンス出版の佐々木一高氏にアドバイス、ご教示をいただいた。ここに書面を借りて御礼申し上げる次第である。

Thomas R. Ward

本書の使用にあたって

　本書は、独学にも、また教室での勉強にも使用できる。歯科診療で外国人患者と接する際の日常的なシチュエーションで、クラウン、根管治療、日本の健康保険などいろいろな説明を、基本的な会話の形で集めたものである。

　本書は12章からなり、それぞれ2つのセクションに分かれている。最初は歯科の1つのトピックを患者にもわかる平易な表現で説明する対話になっている。この対話では専門用語は使っていない。各章の対話の前には場面の説明を簡単にしているが、この中には、歯科医だけが使う専門用語が含まれていることもある。

　第2のセクションには、対話中に出てくる文章を使った、5つの入れ換え練習問題がある。ここに使われている用語は、専門的な性格のもの（う蝕原性の、歯肉切除術など）、患者が理解できる言葉（むし歯、クラウンなど）もある。この練習問題は、文章（構文）をマスターするまで反復練習をするとよいだろう。

　また、本書の最後には、歯科医と患者のコミュニケーションのための、もっとも重要な100語を載せた。これらはすべて歯科用語を特に知らない人にでもわかる言葉である。このような言葉は、患者とのコミュニケーションに欠かせないものなので、対話の勉強を始める前に暗記するのも良いだろう。

　なお、本書を活かすためには、収録した音声を併用して学習することを勧める。

CD（収録音声）の使い方

　本書とセットになったCDには、次のものが収録されている。①各章の英会話すべて、②各章の練習問題の例題すべて、③各章の練習問題の置き換え語句の一部（特に発音が難しいと思われるもの）。

1．各章の英会話を練習する順序と方法

①まず、会話全体をとおして聞いてみる。
②発音と意味がわかったところで、実際に声を出して会話を模倣する。この際、1人が話す度ごとに音声を止め、反復練習をしてみると効果的である。
③次に、自分が対話の一方の役になって、その部分を言ってみる。たとえば、歯科医になったつもりで、音声を止め、歯科医の応答文を言ってみる。次いで音声を再開し、自分の発音、イントネーションが正しいかどうか確認する。この役割練習は、歯科医だけでなく、患者にもなって行うべきである。
④次に双方の役割を1人でこなして、全文を暗記してみる。

2．練習問題の使い方

①例題と語句の置き換わったものを2～3回聞き、声を出して反復練習してみる。
②発音とイントネーションを耳と口が覚えたと思ったら、練習問題の置き換え語句を入れて、次々声を出して練習してみる。その際、発音のわからない語句は、音声で確認する。
③置き換え文章を12まで発音し終わったら、また1まで戻り、置き換えがスムーズに言えるようにする。
　以上、短時間でも繰り返し、納得のいくまで声を出して練習してみよう。

CONTENTS

| まえがき ……………………………………………… | 3 |

| 本書の使用にあたって ……………………………… | 4 |

| CD（収録音声）の使い方 ……………………………… | 5 |

| 第1章　歯内療法の説明 ……………………………… 8
What Is a Root Canal?
根管治療とは何ですか |

| 第2章　歯の全部被覆冠の説明 …………………… 22
What Is a Crown?
クラウンとは何ですか |

| 第3章　歯周病の説明　Ⅰ．診断 …………………… 34
Will All My Teeth Drop Out?
私の歯は全部抜けてしまうのでしょうか |

| 第4章　歯周病の説明　Ⅱ．予後 …………………… 46
What Can You Do to Save My Teeth?
私の歯を救うために、どんなことをしてくださるのですか |

| 第5章　インレーとアマルガム修復の違い ………… 60
What Is an Inlay?
インレーとは何ですか |

第6章　抜歯後の患者への指示 ……………………… 72
Will It Hurt After the Tooth Is Extracted?
歯を抜いた後は痛くなりますか

第7章　乳歯修復の必要性 ………………………………… 86
It's Only a Baby Tooth.
ただの乳歯でしょう

第8章　矯正治療の相談 …………………………………… 98
Why Does My Daughter Need Her Teeth Straightened?
なぜ私の娘は歯並びをなおす必要があるのですか

第9章　ホワイトニングの説明 ……………………… 112
I Want to Have My Teeth Whitened.
歯を白くしたいです

第10章　インプラント治療についてのアドバイス …… 126
What Can I Do about that Missing Tooth?
歯を失った場合、どうすればいいのですか

第11章　外国の歯科保険の使用 …………………… 140
Is the Cost Covered by Insurance?
その治療費は保険がききますか

第12章　外国人に社会保険制度を説明する ………… 152
Can I Use My Social Insurance Card Here?
ここでは、社会健康保険証が使えますか

付録 …………………………………………………… 166
患者とのコミュニケーションで役立つ最重要用語100語

Chapter 1

An explanation of endodontic treatment

What Is a Root Canal?

Although most patients have heard of root canal treatment, many do not know exactly what it means. The following dialogue explains endodontics in terms that the average patient can understand. It is probably a good idea to draw a diagram of a tooth when explaining the treatment.

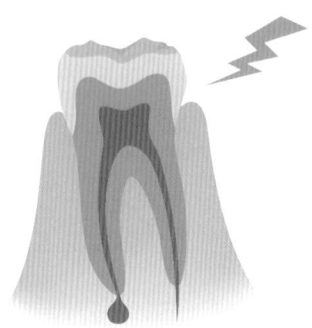

第 1 章

歯内療法の説明

根管治療とは何ですか

　ほとんどの患者は、根管治療という言葉を聞いたことがあるが、それが何であるか正確に知っている人は少ない。以下の対話は普通の患者が理解できる言葉で、歯内療法を説明したものである。治療説明の際、歯の図解を示して説明するのも良いだろう。

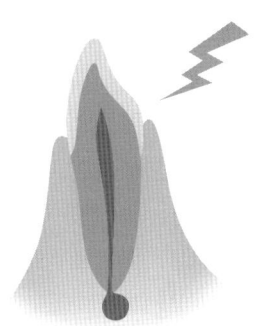

Situation: Mr. Truman, a Canadian businessman, has acute pulpitis in his maxillary right second premolar. He has been told that endodontic treatment is necessary.

Dentist: In order to eliminate the infection and permit restoration of the tooth, it will be necessary to do root canal treatment on your tooth.
Mr. Truman: What is root canal treatment? It sounds terrible.
Dentist: It's really not so bad. First I will give you anesthetic so that there will be no discomfort.
Mr. Truman: I don't like pain.
Dentist: Then I will make a hole through the top of the tooth which leads into the root canal in the center of the root.
Mr. Truman: What is in the canal?
Dentist: There are blood vessels, connective tissue and nerves there.
Mr. Truman: Is it OK to do that?
Dentist: These tissues have become infected due to the large cavity in your tooth. If we do not clean out the infected tissues, the disease will spread into the bone causing more discomfort and perhaps even loss of the tooth.
Mr. Truman: I don't want to lose the tooth.
Dentist: After the infected tissue has all been removed, I will fill the canals with a rubber type substance called gutta percha.
Mr. Truman: Will you finish the treatment today?
Dentist: I want to wait until next week to fill the canals. We

場面：カナダ人ビジネスマン、トルーマン氏は、上顎右側第二小臼歯に急性歯髄炎がある。歯内療法が必要だと告げられたところである。

  歯科医：感染部を取り除いて、歯を修復するには、根管治療が必要でしょうね。

トルーマン：根管治療とは何ですか。こわそうに聞こえますね。
  歯科医：そんなにこわいものじゃありませんよ。痛くないように、まず麻酔をします。
トルーマン：痛いのは苦手ですから……。
  歯科医：それから、歯の一番上に歯の根の中央にある根管にまで届く穴をあけます。

トルーマン：根管には何が入っているんですか。
  歯科医：血管や結合組織や神経が入ってます。

トルーマン：そんなことをして良いんでしょうか。
  歯科医：この組織は大きなむし歯のために、感染を起こしているんです。もし、その感染組織をきれいに取り除かなかったら、骨の方までそれが広がって、もっと痛くなるし、歯を失うことになるかもしれませんよ。

トルーマン：歯は失いたくありません。
  歯科医：感染組織をすべて取り除いた後、ガッタパーチャというガムのような物で根管を詰めます。

トルーマン：治療は今日で終わりますか。
  歯科医：根管を詰めるのは来週まで待ちましょう。脹れと感

should wait until the swelling and infection have gone down.

Mr. Truman: If you take out the nerve, does that mean that I will never get a toothache?

Dentist: That is right. But the tooth can still decay if you do not brush properly.

Mr. Truman: Is it really necessary to have a crown on the tooth after having the root canal?

Dentist: The tooth is very weak due to the decay and the large amount of tooth structure removed while doing the root canal. If a crown is not done, the tooth could actually fracture down the middle.

Mr. Truman: What would happen then?

Dentist: It might have to be extracted.

Mr. Truman: I don't want to lose the tooth. I guess we had better do the crown.

染がおさまるまで待たなければなりませんから。

トルーマン：神経を取り出してしまえば、もう歯痛にはならないってことですか。

歯科医：そうです。でも、きちんと歯を磨かなかったら、むし歯にはなりますよ。

トルーマン：根管治療の後、クラウンは本当に必要ですか。

歯科医：むし歯と、根管治療のため、歯が大きく削りとられるので、とてももろくなります。もし、クラウンをかぶせなかったら、実際にその歯は真ん中で割れてしまう可能性があります。

トルーマン：そうすると、どうなりますか。

歯科医：たぶん、抜歯しなければならないでしょうね。

トルーマン：歯を失いたくはありません。クラウンをかぶせた方が良さそうですね。

Exercises

Ⅰ. Substitute the following expressions in the example dialogue.

— What is <u>root canal treatment</u>? It sounds terrible.
— It's really not so bad.
⟨endodontic treatment⟩
— What is <u>endodontic treatment</u>? It sounds terrible.
— It's really not so bad.

1. periodontal treatment
2. a suture
3. gingivitis
4. gutta percha
5. zinc oxide
6. an apicoectomy
7. amalgam
8. a root fracture
9. a frenectomy
10. xerostomia
11. a skin graft
12. a periodontal probe

Ⅱ. Substitute the following expressions in the example sentence.

In order to eliminate the discomfort, it will be necessary to <u>do a root canal</u>.

練習問題

Ⅰ．例にあげた対話の下線部を次の語句に置き換えなさい。

－<u>根管治療</u>とは何ですか。こわそうに聞こえますね。
－そんなにこわいものじゃありませんよ。
〈歯内療法〉
－<u>歯内療法</u>とは何ですか。こわそうに聞こえますね。
－そんなにこわいものじゃありませんよ。

1. 歯周治療
2. 縫合
3. 歯肉炎
4. ガッタパーチャ
5. 酸化亜鉛
6. 歯根尖切除術
7. アマルガム
8. 歯根破折
9. 小帯切除術
10. 口腔乾燥
11. 皮膚移植
12. 歯周プローブ

Ⅱ．例文の下線部を次の語句に置き換えなさい。

歯痛（不快感）をなくすには、<u>根管治療をする</u>ことが必要でしょう。

⟨see a dentist⟩

In order to eliminate the discomfort, it will be necessary to see a dentist.

1. take medicine
2. treat the tooth
3. see a doctor
4. do an amalgam filling
5. remove the decay
6. take an aspirin
7. stop eating hot foods
8. see an endodontist
9. stop smoking
10. place a suture
11. pull the tooth
12. treat the infection

Ⅲ. Substitute the following expressions in the example sentence.

We should wait until the swelling and infection go down.
⟨tissue heals⟩
We should wait until the tissue heals.

1. symptoms disappear
2. amalgam hardens
3. tooth is extracted
4. hygiene improves

〈歯医者に行く〉
歯痛（不快感）をなくすには、歯医者に行くことが必要でしょう。

1. 薬をのむ
2. 歯を治療する
3. 医者に行く
4. アマルガム充填をする
5. う蝕を除去する
6. アスピリンをのむ
7. 熱い食物を食べるのをやめる
8. 歯内療法専門医に行く
9. 禁煙する
10. 縫合をする
11. 歯を抜く
12. 感染を治療する

Ⅲ．例文の下線部を次の語句に置き換えなさい。

腫れと感染がおさまるまで待たなければなりません。
〈組織が治癒する〉
組織が治癒するまで待たなければなりません。

1. 症状が消える
2. アマルガムが固まる
3. 歯が抜去される
4. 衛生が改善する

5. appliance is finished
6. sutures are removed
7. resin hardens
8. tooth gets better
9. clinic opens
10. central incisor erupts
11. condyle is in the proper location
12. inlay is set

Ⅳ. Substitute the following expressions in the example sentence.

Is it really necessary to have a crown on the tooth?
〈do a root canal〉
Is it really necessary to do a root canal?

1. etch the enamel
2. remove the calculus
3. clean the bur
4. remove the caries
5. use precious metal
6. have an examination
7. brush the gums
8. fill the root canal
9. have interproximal contacts
10. place a core
11. plane the roots
12. probe the pockets

5. 装置が完成する
6. 抜糸する
7. レジンが固まる
8. 歯が良くなる
9. 診療所が開く
10. 中切歯が萌出する
11. 骨頭が正しい位置にいく
12. インレーを装着する

Ⅳ．例文の下線部を次の語句に置き換えなさい。

その歯にクラウンをかぶせるのは、本当に必要ですか。
〈根管治療をする〉
根管治療をするのは、本当に必要ですか。

1. エナメル質をエッチングする
2. 歯石を除去する
3. バーをきれいにする
4. う蝕を除去する
5. 貴金属を使う
6. 診査を受ける
7. 歯ぐきをブラッシングする
8. 根管を詰める
9. 隣接面接触がある
10. コアを装着する
11. ルートプレーニングをする
12. ポケットを測る

Ⅴ. Substitute the following expressions in the example sentence.

I guess we had better <u>do the crown</u>.
〈floss the teeth〉
I guess we had better <u>floss the teeth</u>.

1. cast the crown
2. remove the stain
3. adjust the denture
4. place the rubber dam
5. clean the denture
6. do a flap operation
7. give an injection
8. take an alginate impression
9. consult an orthodontist
10. remove the debris
11. extract the tooth
12. splint the teeth

Ⅴ．例文の下線部を次の語句に置き換えなさい。

クラウンをかぶせた方が良さそうですね。
〈歯をフロスする〉
歯をフロスした方が良さそうですね。

 1. クラウンを鋳造する
 2. ステインを除去する
 3. 義歯を調整する
 4. ラバーダムをはめる
 5. 義歯をきれいにする
 6. 歯肉剥離掻爬術をする
 7. 注射をする
 8. アルギン酸印象をとる
 9. 矯正歯科医に相談する
10. 食べかすを除去する
11. 歯を抜く
12. 歯にスプリントをつける

Chapter 2

An explanation of a full coverage crown

What Is a Crown?

The explanation of crown and bridge treatment is very easy if you draw a simple diagram of the tooth while you are talking with the patient. You can easily gain his confidence and acceptance of your treatment plan using a simple explanation like this.

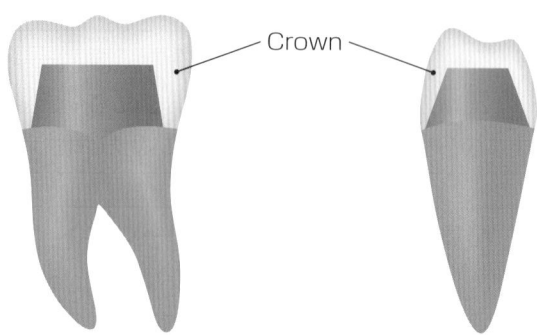

第 2 章

歯の全部被覆冠の説明

クラウンとは何ですか

　クラウンやブリッジ治療は、簡単に歯の図解をすると患者に説明しやすい。このような簡単な説明をすることで、患者の信頼が得られ、治療を受け入れてもらうことができる。

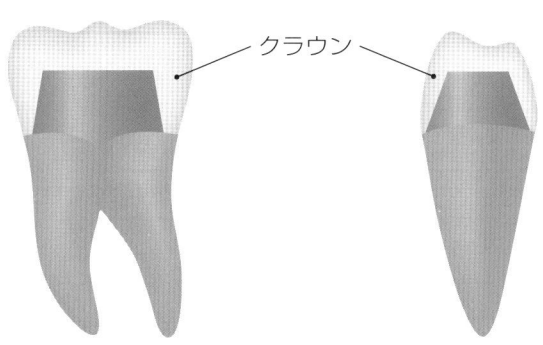
クラウン

Situation: This is a continuation of treatment on the same tooth in the previous dialogue.

Mr. Truman: Can you explain exactly what a crown is?
    Dentist: Sure I would be glad to. The concept is simple if you look at this drawing. This is what the tooth looks like now.
Mr. Truman: There is not very much left. Are you sure you can put a crown on the tooth?
    Dentist: Of course I can. First a small post will be put in the root canal to support the crown.
Mr. Truman: That sounds interesting.
    Dentist: The shape of the post will allow the crown to be one to two millimeters thick all around, like this.
Mr. Truman: Is that post big enough?
    Dentist: It is large enough to hold the crown. We then take an impression and the laboratory technician makes the crown.
Mr. Truman: Is it made of metal?
    Dentist: Since this tooth shows when you smile, I will have the crown made of porcelain.
Mr. Truman: Won't it break?
    Dentist: No. The porcelain is very strong. It is fused to a thin layer of metal which covers the surface of the tooth.
Mr. Truman: Will it look natural?
    Dentist: My technician is very good. The crown will look just like a natural tooth.
Mr. Truman: It is amazing what modern dentistry can do.

場面：前章の対話に出てくる歯の治療の続き。

トルーマン：クラウンとは何ですか、はっきり説明してください。
歯科医：もちろんですとも。この絵をごらんになれば、すぐわかっていただけるでしょう。現在、歯はこのように見えます。
トルーマン：あまり残っているところがありませんね。この歯にクラウンをかぶせることが、本当にできるのですか。
歯科医：もちろんできます。まず、クラウンを支えるため、根管に小さなポストを入れます。
トルーマン：なかなかおもしろいですね。
歯科医：クラウンの厚さが1～2mmになるようなポストの形にします。
トルーマン：そのポストの大きさはそれで良いのですか。
歯科医：クラウンを支えるのには、十分な大きさです。それから印象を取り、歯科技工士がクラウンを作ります。

トルーマン：それは金属でできているんですか。
歯科医：この歯は笑った時に見えますから、ポーセレンで作らせましょう。
トルーマン：割れませんか。
歯科医：いいえ。ポーセレンはとても強いんですよ。歯の表面をおおう金属の薄い層に焼きつけられています。

トルーマン：自然な歯に見えるでしょうか。
歯科医：ここの歯科技工士はとても優秀ですから、クラウンも、自然の歯と同じように見えますよ。
トルーマン：今の歯学は驚異的なことができるのですね。

Exercises

I. Substitute the following expressions in the example dialogue.

−Can you explain exactly what <u>a crown</u> is?
−Sure I would be glad to.
⟨an electron microscope⟩
−Can you explain exactly what <u>an electron microscope</u> is?
−Sure I would be glad to.

1. connective tissue
2. a splint
3. a cyst
4. a ligament
5. a premature contact
6. an onlay
7. braces (are)
8. a bicuspid
9. a local anesthetic
10. a wisdom tooth
11. sealants (are)
12. bruxism

II. Substitute the following expressions in the example sentence.

This is what a <u>tooth</u> looks like.
⟨molar⟩

練習問題

Ⅰ．例にあげた対話の下線部を次の語句に置き換えなさい。

－<u>クラウン</u>とは何ですか、はっきり説明してくださいますか。
－もちろんですとも。
〈電子顕微鏡〉
－<u>電子顕微鏡</u>とは何ですか、はっきり説明してくださいますか。
－もちろんですとも。

1. 結合組織
2. スプリント
3. 嚢胞
4. 靭帯
5. 早期接触
6. オンレー
7. 矯正装置
8. 小臼歯
9. 局部麻酔
10. 智歯
11. シーラント
12. 歯ぎしり

Ⅱ．例文の下線部を次の語句におきかえなさい。

<u>歯</u>はこのように見えます。
〈臼歯〉

This is what a molar looks like.

1. a cusp
2. the ramus
3. a bifurcation
4. a primary tooth
5. a baby tooth
6. the gingiva
7. a crossbite
8. a Hawley appliance
9. a silver filling
10. an anterior tooth
11. calculus
12. a canine

Ⅲ. Substitute the following expressions in the example dialogue.

− Are you sure you can put a crown on the tooth?
− Of course I can.
⟨fill the tooth⟩
− Are you sure you can fill the tooth?
− Of course I can.

1. extract that tooth
2. pull that tooth
3. remove all of the decay
4. make a denture

臼歯はこのように見えます。

1. 咬頭
2. 枝
3. 分岐
4. 乳歯
5. 赤ちゃんの歯
6. 歯肉
7. 交叉咬合
8. ホーレー保定装置
9. 銀の充填物
10. 前歯
11. 歯石
12. 犬歯

Ⅲ．例にあげた対話の下線部を以下の語句におきかえなさい。

－その歯にクラウンをかぶせることは、本当にできるのですか。
－もちろんできますとも。
〈この歯を詰める〉
－その歯を詰めることは、本当にできるのですか。
－もちろんできますとも。

1. この歯を抜く
2. この歯を抜く
3. う蝕をすべて除去する
4. 義歯を作る

5. treat the TMJ problem
6. remove the plaque
7. remove the temporary filling
8. restore the tooth
9. remove the calculus
10. treat this case
11. take an impression
12. etch the enamel

Ⅳ. Substitute the following expressions in the example sentence.

I will have the crown made of <u>porcelain</u>.
⟨gold⟩
I will have the crown made of <u>gold</u>.

1. porcelain fused-to-metal
2. resin
3. quick-curing resin
4. palladium
5. precious metal
6. nonprecious metal
7. a durable material
8. something cheap
9. some type of metal
10. type III gold
11. composite resin
12. type II gold

5. 顎関節の問題を治療する
6. プラークを除去する
7. 暫間的な充填物を除去する
8. この歯を修復する
9. 歯石を除去する
10. この症例を治療する
11. 印象を採る
12. エナメル質をエッチングする

Ⅳ. 例文の下線部を次の語句に置き換えなさい。

クラウンを<u>ポーセレン</u>で作らせましょう。
〈金〉
クラウンを<u>金</u>で作らせましょう。

1. 金属焼付ポーセレン
2. レジン
3. 即時重合レジン
4. パラジウム
5. 貴金属
6. 卑金属
7. 耐久性のある材料
8. 何か安いもの
9. ある種の金属
10. タイプⅢの金
11. コンポジットレジン
12. タイプⅡの金

Ⅴ. Substitute the following expressions in the example sentence.

It is amazing what modern dentistry can do.
〈dental hygienists〉
It is amazing what dental hygienists can do.

1. modern science
2. dental science
3. my dentist
4. dental technicians
5. periodontists
6. orthodontists
7. orthodontic appliances
8. gum surgery
9. good oral hygiene
10. brushing
11. a good technician
12. my dental hygienist

Ⅴ．例文の下線部を次の語句に置き換えなさい。

<u>今の歯学</u>は驚異的なことができるのですね。
〈歯科衛生士〉
<u>歯科衛生士</u>は驚異的なことができるのですね。

1. 近代科学
2. 歯学
3. 私の歯科医
4. 歯科技工士
5. 歯周病専門医
6. 矯正歯科医
7. 矯正装置
8. 歯肉手術
9. 良い口腔衛生
10. ブラッシング
11. 良い技工士
12. 私の歯科衛生士

Chapter 3

An explanation of periodontal disease
Part I : The diagnosis

Will All My Teeth Drop Out?

Most patients have heard of periodontal disease but few of them realize how serious it can be. Showing the patient the pocket probing depths which you have charted is a good way to impress upon him the seriousness of his disease. A simple drawing of the tooth, pocket and periodontal membrane will aid in the explanation.

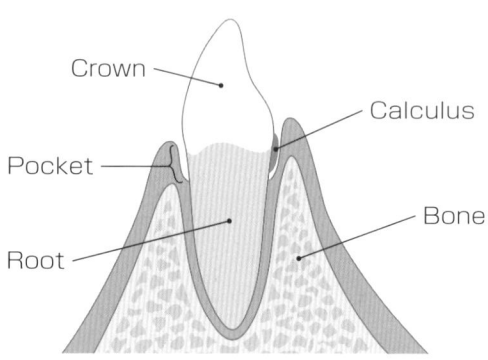

第3章

歯周病の説明　I. 診断

私の歯は全部抜けてしまうのでしょうか

　多くの患者は、歯周病について聞いたことはあるが、それがどんなに重大なものか理解している人は少ない。チャートに書き入れたポケットの深さを患者に見せることは、疾患の重大さを印象づける良い方法である。歯、ポケット、歯周粘膜を簡単に描くのも説明の助けになるだろう。

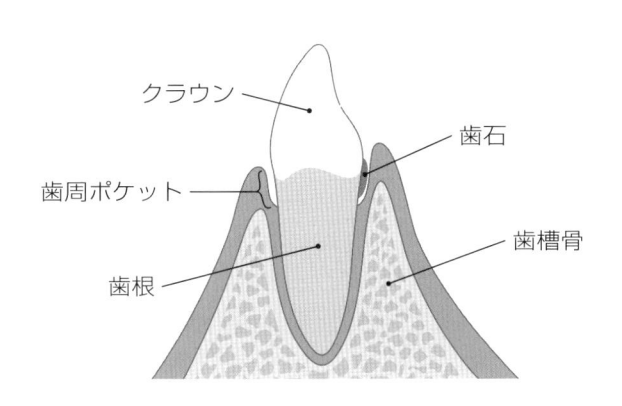

- クラウン
- 歯石
- 歯周ポケット
- 歯槽骨
- 歯根

Situation: Mrs. Boster, a 47-year-old housewife from New Zealand, has been neglecting a serious periodontal condition for several years. The dentist is explaining why treatment is necessary and what must be done.

Mrs. Boster: What do all those pocket depths mean? Will all my teeth drop out?
Dentist: This diagram of the tooth should help you understand the situation. A pocket around the tooth of two to three millimeters is normal.
Mrs. Boster: Doesn't food get caught in the pocket?
Dentist: Yes, but when it is only a few millimeters deep, it can easily be cleaned with a toothbrush.
Mrs. Boster: What happens when it is deeper?
Dentist: A pocket depth of 4 or 5 millimeters indicates gum disease. At this depth, it cannot be adequately cleaned by brushing and flossing.
Mrs. Boster: What happens then?
Dentist: Eventually plaque and calculus build up in the pocket. The bacteria produce acid which destroys the supporting tissues around the root, and the pocket gets deeper.
Mrs. Boster: That sounds pretty bad. Does the tooth fall out?
Dentist: Not yet. But eventually it becomes loose. When the pockets exceed 7 millimeters, the situation becomes quite serious. There is bleeding from the gums and unless treatment is done, the tooth will be lost.
Mrs. Boster: I don't want that to happen.

場面：47歳のニュージーランド人主婦、ボスター夫人は、数年間、危険な歯周状態を無視してきた。歯科医は、なぜ治療が必要か、何をしなければならないかを説明している。

ボスター：このポケットの探さは、どういう意味ですか。私の歯は全部抜けてしまうのでしょうか。
歯科医：この歯の図を見ると、どういう状態か理解しやすくなると思います。歯の周りの2～3mmのポケットは正常です。
ボスター：食べ物がポケットの中に入りませんか。
歯科医：はい、入ります。しかしポケットの深さが2～3mmなら、歯ブラシで簡単にきれいにできるでしょう。
ボスター：もしもっと深いと、どうなるのですか。
歯科医：ポケットの探さが4～5mmということは、歯ぐきの病気を示しています。この探さではブラッシングやフロスでは完全にきれいにすることができません。
ボスター：そうするとどうなりますか。
歯科医：結局、プラークと歯石がポケットの中に増えてきます。バクテリアが根の周りの支持組織を破壊する酸を出し、ポケットはますます深くなっていくんです。

ボスター：それは大変ですわね。歯は抜けてしまうんでしょうか。
歯科医：いえ、まだです。でも、結局ぐらぐらになってしまいますよ。ポケットが7mmを越えると、状況は非常に危険になります。歯肉から出血もしますし、治療しなければ、その歯は抜けてしまうでしょう。
ボスター：そんなことになるのはいやですわ。

Exercises

Ⅰ. Substitute the following expressions in the example sentence.

Most patients have heard of periodontal disease.
〈flap operations〉
Most patients have heard of flap operations.

1. space maintainers
2. cancer
3. tooth decay
4. plaque
5. oral surgery
6. wisdom teeth
7. crowns
8. modern dentistry
9. porcelain
10. dentures
11. sutures
12. fluoride

Ⅱ. Substitute the following expressions in the example sentence.

She has been neglecting a serious periodontal condition for several years.
〈her teeth〉

練習問題

Ⅰ．例文の下線部を次の語句に置き換えなさい。

多くの患者は、歯周疾患について聞いたことがある。
〈歯肉剥離掻爬術〉
多くの患者は歯肉剥離掻爬術について聞いたことがある。

1. 保隙装置
2. がん
3. むし歯
4. プラーク
5. 口腔外科
6. 智歯
7. クラウン
8. 近代歯学
9. ポーセレン
10. 義歯
11. 縫合
12. フッ化物

Ⅱ．例文の下線部を次の語句に置き換えなさい。

彼女は、数年間、危険な歯周状態を無視してきた。

〈彼女の歯〉

She has been neglecting her teeth for several years.

1. her mouth
2. her health
3. the cavity
4. her plaque control
5. seeing a dentist
6. to seek orthodontic treatment
7. a heart condition
8. the periodontitis
9. the pain
10. the tumor
11. dental care for her children
12. her responsibilities

Ⅲ. Substitute the following expressions in the example sentence.

This diagram should help you understand the situation.
⟨explanation⟩
This explanation should help you understand the situation.

1. picture
2. graph
3. book
4. idea
5. demonstration
6. X-ray

彼女は、数年間、自分の歯（の手入れ）を怠ってきた。

1. 彼女の口（の手入れ）
2. 彼女の健康（の維持）
3. むし歯（への治療）
4. プラークコントロール
5. 歯医者に行くこと
6. 矯正治療をする努力
7. 心臓病（についての注意）
8. 歯周炎（についての注意）
9. 痛み（を治療すること）
10. 腫瘍（を治療すること）
11. 子どもの歯の手入れ
12. 彼女の責任（を果たすこと）

Ⅲ．例文の下線部を次の語句に置き換えなさい。

この図を見れば、どういう状態か理解しやすくなると思います。
〈説明〉
この説明で、どういう状態か理解しやすくなると思います。

1. 絵
2. グラフ
3. 本
4. 考え
5. 実演
6. エックス線写真

7. pamphlet
8. study model
9. plaster model
10. wax denture model
11. videotape
12. simple diagram

Ⅳ. Substitute the following expressions in the example sentence.

A pocket depth of 4 or 5 millimeters indicates gum disease.
⟨periodontal disease⟩
A pocket depth of 4 or 5 millimeters indicates periodontal disease.

1. periodontal problems
2. reversible periodontitis
3. a need for root planing
4. a need for better oral hygiene
5. poor oral health
6. potential for bleeding gingiva
7. the beginning of gum disease
8. poor brushing
9. the need for interproximal brushing
10. problems with the gums
11. a need for treatment
12. a need for curettage

7. パンフレット
 8. スタディモデル
 9. 石膏模型
10. 義歯のワックス模型
11. ビデオテープ
12. 簡単な図

Ⅳ．例文の下線部を次の語句に置き換えなさい。

ポケットの探さが4〜5mmということは、歯ぐきの病気を示しています。
〈歯周疾患〉
ポケットの探さが4〜5mmということは、歯周疾患を示しています。

 1. 歯周の問題
 2. 治療可能な歯周炎
 3. ルートプレーニングが必要であること
 4. もっと良い口腔衛生が必要であること
 5. 不健康な口腔
 6. 歯肉出血の可能性がある
 7. 歯ぐきの病気のはじまり
 8. 不適切なブラッシング
 9. 歯間ブラシが必要であること
10. 歯ぐきの問題
11. 治療が必要であること
12. 掻爬が必要であること

V. Substitute the following expressions in the example dialogue.

－Unless treatment is carried out, the <u>tooth will be lost</u>.
－I don't want that to happen.
〈problem will get worse〉
－Unless treatment is carried out, the <u>problem will get worse</u>.
－I don't want that to happen.

1. tooth will ache
2. gums will bleed
3. periodontal condition will worsen
4. condition will not get better
5. patient will be dissatisfied
6. child will have more problems
7. tooth will get worse
8. infection will spread
9. decay will reach the pulp
10. tooth will become mobile
11. periodontal pockets will worsen
12. periodontal ligament will be destroyed

Ⅴ．例にあげた対話の下線部を次の語句に置き換えなさい。

－治療しなければ、その歯は抜けてしまうでしょう。
－そんなことになるのはいやです。
〈問題がいっそう悪くなるでしょう〉
－治療しなければ、その問題はいっそう悪くなるでしょう。
－そんなことになるのはいやです。

 1. 歯が痛くなるでしょう
 2. 歯肉から出血するでしょう
 3. 歯周状態はもっと悪くなるでしょう
 4. 状態は良くならないでしょう
 5. 患者は不満足でしょう
 6. 子どもはもっと問題を持つことになるでしょう
 7. 歯がいっそう悪くなるでしょう
 8. 感染が広がるでしょう
 9. う蝕が歯髄にまで達するでしょう
10. 歯が動揺するようになるでしょう
11. 歯周ポケットがもっと悪くなるでしょう
12. 歯根膜が破壊されるでしょう

Chapter 4

An explanation of periodontal disease
Part II : The prognosis

What Can You Do to Save My Teeth?

Since periodontal treatment is expensive and time consuming, it is very important that the patient understands why it is necessary and what the prognosis will be for maintaining his teeth. It is essential to tell him that the treatment will be of little benefit unless he practices thorough oral hygiene.

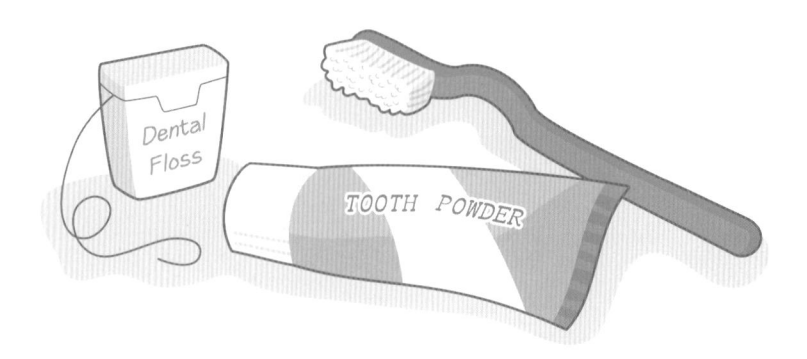

第 4 章

歯周病の説明　Ⅱ．予後

私の歯を救うために、どんなことをしてくださるのですか

　歯周治療は高額であり、時間もかかるので、なぜ治療が必要か、歯を保つための予後はどうかを、患者がよく理解することが大切である。もし患者が、徹底的に口腔衛生を実行しなければ、治療そのものはほとんど役に立たないと告げることが非常に大切である。

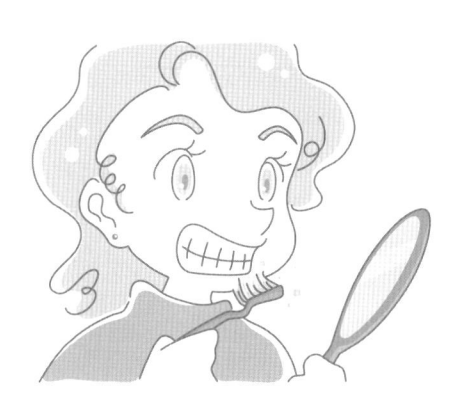

Situation: This is a continuation of the previous dialogue.

Mrs. Boster: What treatment can you do to save my teeth?

Dentist: It is important that you understand that 90% of the treatment must be done by you.
Mrs. Boster: How can I do that? I am not a dentist.

Dentist: You don't need to be a dentist. All you have to do is thoroughly brush and floss your teeth every day.
Mrs. Boster: That might be difficult.
Dentist: If you cannot keep your teeth clean, no amount of gum surgery will do any good.
Mrs. Boster: Well, I will do my best. But what are you going to do?
Dentist: Our goal is to get all of the pockets down to within two or three millimeters.
Mrs. Boster: How will we do that?
Dentist: First, you must brush and floss every day.
Mrs. Boster: I thought you would say that.
Dentist: Then the hygienist will do a thorough cleaning, removing all the calculus and plaque from the teeth. She will also give you instructions on brushing and flossing.
Mrs. Boster: I was afraid you would complain about my brushing.
Dentist: With the cleaning and your home care, the pockets may be reduced one or two millimeters.
Mrs. Boster: That's good. Then you won't have to do surgery.

場面：前章の会話の続き

ボスター：私の歯を救うために、どんなことをしてくださるのですか。
歯科医：大事なのは、治療の90％はあなた自身がするということを知っていただくことです。
ボスター：どうすればいいんですか。私、歯医者じゃありませんし……。
歯科医：歯医者でなくてもかまいません。毎日、徹底的に歯を磨き、フロスさえすれば良いのです。
ボスター：なかなか難しそうですね。
歯科医：歯にプラークがつかないようにしておけないのなら、歯ぐきの手術をしても何にもなりませんよ。
ボスター：じゃあ、できる限りやってみます。でも、先生はどういうことをしてくださるんですの。
歯科医：目的は、すべてのポケットを2～3mmの探さまでにすることです。
ボスター：どのようにするのですか。
歯科医：まず、毎日ブラッシングとフロスをしていただきます。
ボスター：そうおっしゃると思ってましたわ。
歯科医：それから、歯科衛生士が徹底的にクリーニングをして、歯石やプラークをすべて取ります。また、ブラッシングやフロスの指導もします。

ボスター：私のブラッシングが悪いとおっしゃるだろうと思ってました。
歯科医：クリーニングとホームケアで、ポケットは1～2mm浅くなることもあります。
ボスター：なるほど。そうすると手術する必要がなくなりますね。

Dentist: You have several pockets in the 6 to 8 millimeter range. They will most likely require some type of surgery.

Mrs. Boster: I don't want to do surgery if it is not necessary.

Dentist: Before gum surgery is done, I will do a deep cleaning of the pockets which is called root planing and curettage. This will remove the calculus and diseased tissue from deep within the pockets.

Mrs. Boster: Will that help?

Dentist: That might reduce the pockets another millimeter if we are lucky.

Mrs. Boster: And if there are still deep pockets, what do we do?

Dentist: Then I will have to do surgery which removes some of the gum tissue from around the teeth. But keep in mind the more you brush, the less I will have to cut.

Mrs. Boster: I'm going to brush as hard as I can.

歯科医：いくつかのポケットは、6〜8mmあります。おそらく、そういうものには、何らかの手術が必要でしょう。

ボスター：不必要な手術はしたくありませんわ。
歯科医：手術の前に、ルートプレーニングと、掻爬という、ポケットの中の深いクリーニングをします。これで、ポケットの中の歯石と病的組織を取り除くわけです。

ボスター：それが役に立つんですか。
歯科医：うまくいけば、それでポケットが1mmほど減るかもしれません。
ボスター：それでもポケットが深いと、どうするのですか。
歯科医：その時は、歯の周りから歯肉組織を少し取り除く手術をしなければなりません。でも、歯を磨けば磨くほど、私が切り取る部分も少なくなると覚えておいてください。
ボスター：できる限り一生懸命磨きます。

Exercises

I. Substitute the following expressions in the example sentence.

It is essential to tell the patient.
⟨brush thoroughly⟩
It is essential to brush thoroughly.

1. use floss
2. use an interproximal brush
3. visit the dentist every six months
4. take care of your teeth
5. have a clean mouth
6. maintain healthy gum tissues
7. have the teeth cleaned
8. listen to your dentist
9. follow your hygienist's instructions
10. inform the patient
11. curettage the periodontal pockets
12. maintain the health of the periodontal tissues

II. Substitute the following expressions in the example sentence.

What can you do to save my teeth?
⟨improve my health⟩
What can you do to improve my health?

練習問題

Ⅰ．例文の下線部を次の語句に置き換えなさい。

患者に告げることが非常に大切である。
〈徹底的に磨く〉
徹底的に磨くことが非常に大切である。

1. フロスを使う
2. 歯間ブラシを使う
3. 6ヵ月ごとに歯医者に行く
4. 歯の手入れをする
5. きれいな口を持つ
6. 健康的な歯ぐきを維持する
7. 歯をクリーニングしてもらう
8. 歯科医の言うことを聞く
9. 歯科衛生士の指導に従う
10. 患者に知らせる
11. 歯周ポケットを搔爬する
12. 歯周組織の健康を維持する

Ⅱ．例文の下線部を次の語句に置き換えなさい。

私の歯を救うために、どんなことをしてくださるのですか。
〈私の健康を改善する〉
私の健康を改善するために、どんなことをしてくださるのですか。

1. improve my smile
2. fix my dentures
3. treat the problem
4. save the tooth
5. eliminate the pain
6. treat the tooth
7. restore the tooth
8. correct the malocclusion
9. restore the occlusion
10. remove the stain
11. eliminate the calculus
12. treat the periodontal condition

Ⅲ. Substitute the following expressions in the example sentence.

All you have to do is brush your teeth every day.
〈clean your teeth〉
All you have to do is clean your teeth every day.

1. take care of your teeth
2. floss your teeth
3. brush your tongue
4. eat nutritious food
5. maintain your oral hygiene
6. use an interproximal brush
7. remove the plaque
8. use an electric toothbrush

1. 私の笑顔を良くする
 2. 私の義歯を修理する
 3. その問題を治療する
 4. その歯が抜けないようにする
 5. 痛みを取る
 6. その歯を治療する
 7. その歯を修復する
 8. 不正咬合を治す
 9. 咬合を修復する
10. ステインを除去する
11. 歯石を取る
12. 歯周状態を治療する

Ⅲ．例文の下線部を次の語句に置き換えなさい。

毎日、歯を磨きさえすれば良いのです。
〈歯をきれいにする〉
毎日、歯をきれいにしさえすれば良いのです。

1. 歯の手入れをする
2. 歯をフロスする
3. 舌をブラッシングする
4. 栄養のある食べ物を食べる
5. 口腔衛生を実行する
6. 歯間ブラシを使う
7. プラークを除去する
8. 電動ブラシを使う

9. brush the occlusal surfaces
10. be aware of your dental health
11. take care of your health
12. eliminate the plaque

Ⅳ. Substitute the following expressions in the example sentence.

The more you brush, the less I will have to cut.
〈floss〉
The more you floss, the less I will have to cut.

1. brush your teeth
2. take care of your teeth
3. eliminate plaque
4. use the toothbrush
5. clean your teeth
6. use the interproximal brush
7. eliminate the pockets
8. care for your gums
9. take care of your oral health
10. try
11. care for your teeth
12. floss your teeth

9. 咬合面を磨く
10. 歯の健康に気をつける
11. 体を大切にする
12. プラークを取る

Ⅳ．例文の下線部を次の語句に置き換えなさい。

<u>磨けば磨くほど</u>、私が切り取る部分も少なくなります。
〈フロスする〉
<u>フロスすればするほど</u>、私が切り取る部分も少なくなります。

1. 歯を磨く
2. 歯を大切にする
3. プラークを取る
4. 歯ブラシを使う
5. 歯をきれいにする
6. 歯間ブラシを使う
7. ポケットをなくす
8. 歯ぐきの手入れをする
9. 口腔衛生を大切にする
10. 努力する
11. 歯の手入れをする
12. 歯をフロスする

Ⅴ. Substitute the following expressions in the example sentence.

I am going to brush as hard as I can.
⟨floss⟩
I am going to floss as hard as I can.

1. work
2. try
3. brush and floss
4. clean my teeth
5. try to brush
6. try to floss
7. remove plaque
8. clean the teeth
9. use the toothbrush
10. use the interproximal brush
11. try to brush and floss
12. try to clean my teeth

Ⅴ．例文の下線部を次の語句に置き換えなさい。

できる限り一生懸命磨きます。
〈フロスする〉
できる限り一生懸命フロスします。

1. 働く
2. 努力する
3. ブラッシングとフロスをする
4. 歯をきれいにする
5. 磨こうとする
6. フロスしようとする
7. プラークを除去する
8. 歯をきれいにする
9. 歯ブラシを使う
10. 歯間ブラシを使う
11. ブラッシングとフロスをしようとする
12. 歯をきれいにしようとする

Chapter 5

The difference between inlays
and amalgam restorations

What Is an Inlay?

Since inlays are rarely done in America and Europe, many foreign patients are surprised to learn that it takes two visits to complete a simple filling. The following explains the difference between inlays and amalgams.

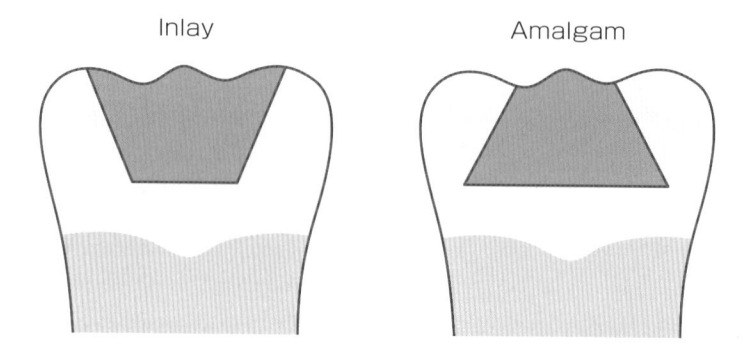

Inlay   Amalgam

第 5 章

インレーとアマルガム修復の違い

インレーとは何ですか

　欧米では、インレーはあまり使われないので、1つの簡単な充填に2回来院が必要だと言うと、驚く外国人患者が多い。以下は、インレーとアマルガムの違いの説明である。

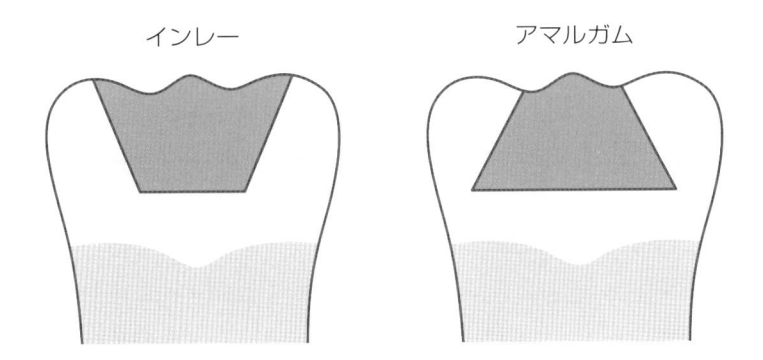

インレー　　　　　　アマルガム

Situation: Mr. Chevalier, a Frenchman, came to the office to have one small class II carious lesion restored. He was surprised that the treatment would take two visits.

Mr. Chevalier: I would like to have that small cavity filled today. I am leaving for Paris tomorrow.

Dentist: I am afraid I will not be able to finish it today. It takes a few days to make the inlay in the laboratory.

Mr. Chevalier: What is an inlay?

Dentist: An inlay is a casting which is placed into the tooth after the tooth has been prepared by removing the decay.

Mr. Chevalier: My dentist in Paris always completed fillings in one day. Why can't you?

Dentist: Your dentist used amalgam. It is a mixture of silver and mercury which is packed into the tooth while soft. It hardens completely in a few hours.

Mr. Chevalier: Don't you have amalgam?

Dentist: Yes, I do. However, this cavity is too large to fill with amalgam.

Mr. Chevalier: I will be away on business for two weeks and would like to have the tooth taken care of before I leave.

Dentist: I will place a temporary filling in the tooth which you can use until you come back to Japan.

Mr. Chevalier: That would be very nice.

Dentist: I will place the inlay when you return.

Mr. Chevalier: Thank you.

場面：フランス人、シェバリエ氏は、小さなクラスⅡのう蝕を修復してもらうため来院。治療に2回の来院が必要だというので驚いた。

シェバリエ：今日は、小さなむし歯を詰めていただきたいのですが。明日パリに発ちますので。
歯科医：残念ながら、今日それを終えることはできないと思います。ラボでインレーを作るのに2〜3日かかりますから。
シェバリエ：インレーとは何ですか。
歯科医：インレーというのは、歯からう蝕をとった後、そこに入れる鋳造物のことです。

シェバリエ：パリの私の歯医者は、いつも1日で詰めてくれましたがね。どうして、ここではできないんですか。
歯科医：あなたの歯医者はアマルガムを使ったのです。銀と水銀の合金で、柔らかいうちに歯に詰めるもので、それは2〜3時間で完全に固まります。
シェバリエ：先生は、アマルガムがないのですか。
歯科医：いえ、あります。しかし、アマルガム充填をするには、穴が大きすぎますね。
シェバリエ：仕事で2週間留守しますし、発つ前に歯の方をちゃんとしておきたいのです。
歯科医：それでは、歯に一時しのぎの詰めものをしておきましょう。日本にお帰りになるまでもつはずです。
シェバリエ：それがよさそうですね。
歯科医：お帰りになったら、インレーをやりましょう。
シェバリエ：ありがとうございます。

Exercises

Ⅰ. Substitute the following expressions in the example sentence.

What is the difference between <u>an inlay and amalgam</u>?
⟨amalgam and composite resin⟩
What is the difference between <u>amalgam and composite resin</u>?

1. insurance and private treatment
2. gold and amalgam
3. precious and nonprecious metal
4. dentin and enamel
5. cementum and dentin
6. a molar and a premolar
7. dentin and bone
8. a crown and an inlay
9. composite resin and silicate cement
10. calculus and plaque
11. a third molar and a wisdom tooth
12. periodontitis and gingivitis

Ⅱ. Substitute the following expressions in the example sentence.

He was surprised that the treatment <u>would take two visits</u>.
⟨would take so much time⟩
He was surprised that the treatment <u>would take so much time</u>.

練習問題

Ⅰ．例文の下線部を次の語句に置き換えなさい。

インレーとアマルガムの違いは何ですか。
〈アマルガムとコンポジットレジン〉
アマルガムとコンポジットレジンの違いは何ですか。

1. 保険診療と自由診療
2. 金とアマルガム
3. 貴金属と卑金属
4. 象牙質とエナメル質
5. セメント質と象牙質
6. 臼歯と小臼歯
7. 象牙質と骨
8. クラウンとインレー
9. コンポジットレジンと珪酸セメント
10. 歯石とプラーク
11. 第三大臼歯と智歯
12. 歯周炎と歯肉炎

Ⅱ．例文の下線部を次の語句に置き換えなさい。

彼は、治療に2回の来院が必要だというので驚いた。
〈そんなに時間がかかる〉
彼は、治療がそんなに時間がかかるというので驚いた。

1. was expensive
2. was not expensive
3. could be paid by insurance
4. took so long
5. was finished
6. was painless
7. was so difficult
8. would be completed soon
9. required anesthetic
10. required two visits
11. required so much time
12. was so simple

Ⅲ. Substitute the following expressions in the example sentence.

I will be away on business for two weeks and would like to have the tooth taken care of before I leave.
〈the treatment〉
I will be away on business for two weeks and would like to have the treatment taken care of before I leave.

1. the filling
2. the extraction
3. the crown
4. the infection
5. the gum surgery
6. the root canal treatment

1. 高価だ
2. 高価でない
3. 保険でできる
4. そんなに長くかかる
5. 終了した
6. 痛みがない
7. そんなに難しい
8. もうすぐ終わる
9. 麻酔がいる
10. 2回来院がいる
11. そんなに時間がいる
12. そんなに簡単だ

Ⅲ．例文の下線部を次の語句に置き換えなさい。

仕事で2週間留守しますし、発つ前に歯の方をちゃんとしておきたいのです。
〈処置〉
仕事で2週間留守しますし、発つ前に処置をちゃんとしておきたいのです。

1. 充填
2. 抜歯
3. クラウン
4. 感染（の治療）
5. 歯ぐきの手術
6. 根管治療

7. all dental treatment
8. the inlay
9. my temporomandibular joint treatment
10. my teeth
11. the decay
12. my hygiene appointments

Ⅳ. Substitute the following expressions in the example sentence.

I am afraid I will not be able to finish it today.
⟨see you⟩
I am afraid I will not be able to see you.

1. do the treatment
2. complete the root canal treatment today
3. finish
4. save the tooth
5. do periodontal treatment
6. fix the tooth
7. treat this condition
8. take an X-ray
9. complete the inlay today
10. place the crown today
11. extract the tooth
12. do the diagnosis

7. 歯の治療を全部
8. インレー
9. 顎関節の治療
10. 私の歯
11. むし歯
12. 衛生指導の予約

Ⅳ．例文の下線部を次の語句に置き換えなさい。

残念ながら、今日それを終えることはできないと思います。
〈あなたに会う〉
残念ながら、あなたに会うことはできないと思います。

1. 治療をする
2. 今日根管治療を終える
3. 終える
4. その歯が抜けないようにする
5. 歯周治療をする
6. 歯をなおす
7. この状態を治療する
8. エックス線写真を撮る
9. 今日インレーを完成する
10. 今日クラウンを装着する
11. その歯を抜く
12. 診断をする

Ⅴ. Substitute the following expressions in the example dialogue.

- If you like, I suppose I could do an amalgam filling.
- I would appreciate that very much.

⟨complete the restoration⟩

- If you like, I suppose I could complete the restoration.
- I would appreciate that very much.

1. extract the tooth
2. place the crown
3. do the gum surgery
4. complete the treatment
5. do the root planing
6. do the cleaning
7. bleach the tooth
8. excise the lesion
9. take the X-ray
10. make the crown
11. evaluate the periodontal condition
12. probe the pockets

Ⅴ．例にあげた対話の下線部を次の語句に置き換えなさい。

－もしお望みなら、アマルガム充填をすることもできますが……。
－そうしていただけるとたいへんありがたいです。
〈修復を仕上げる〉
－もしお望みなら、修復を完成することもできますが……。
－そうしていただけるとたいへんありがたいです。

 1．歯を抜く
 2．クラウンを装着する
 3．歯ぐきの手術をする
 4．治療を完成する
 5．ルートプレーニングをする
 6．クリーニングをする
 7．歯を漂白する
 8．病巣部を切除する
 9．エックス線写真を撮る
10．クラウンを作る
11．歯周状態を評価する
12．ポケットを測る

Chapter 6

Instructions for the patient following the extraction of a tooth

Will It Hurt After the Tooth Is Extracted?

The patient should be given proper home-care instructions following the extraction of a tooth. This is important to minimize pain and to prevent a dry socket infection.

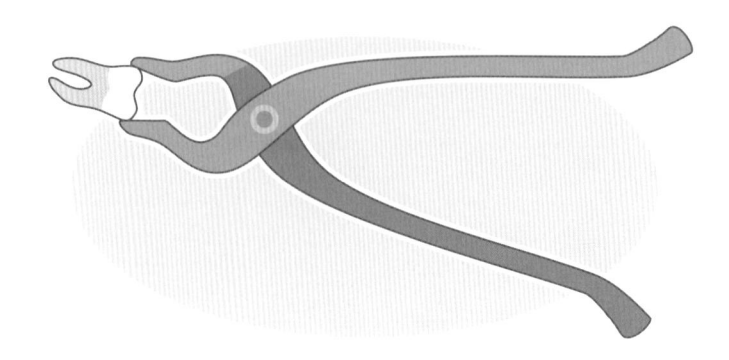

第 6 章

抜歯後の患者への指示

歯を抜いた後は
痛くなりますか

　患者には、抜歯後どんなホームケアをするべきか適切な指示を与えるべきである。これは、痛みを最小限におさえ、ドライソケット感染を防ぐため重要なことである。

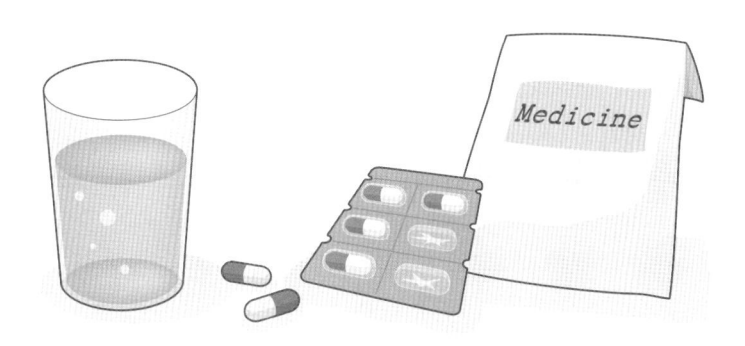

Situation: Ms. Perry, an exchange student from England, has come to the office to have an impacted mandibular third molar extracted. The dentist is giving her postoperative instructions.

Ms. Perry: Will it hurt after the tooth is extracted?
   Dentist: It may be a bit uncomfortable, especially for the first day or two.
Ms. Perry: Should I stay in bed?
   Dentist: That won't be necessary. But you should not do strenuous exercise as it might make the condition worse.
Ms. Perry: Will you give me a pain killer?
   Dentist: Yes. Here is some medicine to relieve the discomfort. Take it only if you need it. You might want to take one tablet before going to bed tonight.
Ms. Perry: How about eating? May I eat today?
   Dentist: You may eat if you like. But don't take foods which are spicy or hot. Soft foods like mashed potatoes or soup would be better for the first day or two.
Ms. Perry: Will there be much bleeding after I return home?
   Dentist: The wound may bleed a small amount each hour for the rest of the day. If bleeding is a problem, put one of these cotton rolls over the wound and bite down on it for 20 minutes. If the bleeding continues, call me. Here is my home phone number as well as the office number.
Ms. Perry: Thank you. I am sure there will be no problem, but it

場面：イギリス人交換留学生ペリーさんは、埋伏第三大臼歯を抜歯してもらうため来院。歯科医は彼女に術後の指示を与えている。

ペリー：歯を抜いた後は痛くなりますか。
歯科医：特に最初の1日か2日は、ちょっと不快感があるかもしれません。
ペリー：ベッドで寝ていた方がいいですか。
歯科医：それは必要ないでしょう。でも、はげしい運動はしない方が良いですよ。状態がもっと悪くなるかもしれませんからね。
ペリー：痛みどめはくださいますか。
歯科医：ええ。ここに不快感を和らげる薬がありますから、必要な時だけのんでください。今夜寝る前に、一錠のみたくなるかもしれません。
ペリー：食事はどうでしょう。今日は、食べてもよろしいですか。
歯科医：食べたいなら食べてもけっこうです。でも、スパイシーなものや、熱い食べ物はとらないように。マッシュポテトや、スープなど軟らかい食べ物が、はじめの1～2日は良いでしょう。
ペリー：家に帰った後たくさん出血するでしょうか。
歯科医：今日1日は、傷口から1時間に少しほどの出血があるかもしれません。もし出血が困るほどなら、このコットンロールを傷口にあてて、20分ほど噛んでいてください。もし、出血し続けるようなら、私に電話してください。ここに診療所と自宅の電話番号が書いてありますから。

ペリー：ありがとうございます。きっと問題はないと思いますけ

is nice to have your number just in case.

Dentist: Also, I am giving you antibiotics for three days. Take one tablet every six hours. This is to prevent an infection from occurring.

Ms. Perry: Should I take the antibiotics even if there is no pain?

Dentist: Yes. It is very important to take all of the antibiotics. This is to help prevent an infection.

Ms. Perry: When should I come back to your office?

Dentist: If there is no discomfort and the healing is good, you need not return here. If you have a bad taste in your mouth or discomfort after a few days, come back immediately.

Ms. Perry: Thank you.

ど、万一の時のために、先生の電話番号を持っていると良いですものね。
歯科医：それに、3日分の抗生物質を出しておきますから、6時間ごとに1錠のんでください。これは、感染が起こるのを防ぐためです。
ペリー：痛くなくても、抗生物質はのんだ方がいいのですか。
歯科医：そうです。抗生物質は全部のみきってしまうことが大切ですよ。これは感染を防ぐのを助けるわけですからね。
ペリー：次はいつ来院したら良いでしょうか。
歯科医：もし、不快感もなく、治っているようなら再来院する必要はありません。もし口の中で変な味がしたり、2〜3日後に不快感があるようなら、すぐに再来院してください。

ペリー：ありがとうございました。

Exercises

Ⅰ. Substitute the following expressions in the example dialogue.

- Should I <u>stay in bed</u>?
- That won't be necessary.

⟨see a doctor⟩
- Should I <u>see a doctor</u>?
- That won't be necessary.

1. have the tooth extracted
2. see an oral surgeon
3. take antibiotics
4. take a pain killer
5. take vitamins
6. have a blood test
7. stop eating hard candy
8. go to bed
9. take medicine
10. have surgery
11. take aspirin
12. go to the hospital

Ⅱ. Substitute the following expressions in the example sentence.

The patient should be given proper instructions on what to do following <u>the extraction of a tooth.</u>

練習問題

Ⅰ．例にあげた対話の下線部を次の語句に置き換えなさい。

－<u>ベッドで寝ていた</u>方がいいですか。
－それは必要ないでしょう。
〈医者に行く〉
－<u>医者に行った</u>方がいいですか。
－それは必要ないでしょう。

1. 歯を抜いてもらう
2. 口腔外科医に見せた
3. 抗生物質をのむ
4. 痛みどめをのむ
5. ビタミンをとる
6. 血液検査を受ける
7. 固いキャンディを食べるのをやめる
8. 寝る
9. 薬をのむ
10. 手術を受ける
11. アスピリンをのむ
12. 病院に行く

Ⅱ．例文の下線部を次の語句に置き換えなさい。

患者には、<u>抜歯</u>後何をするべきか適切な指示を与えるべきである。

⟨periodontal surgery⟩

The patient should be given proper instructions on what to do following periodontal surgery.

1. dental treatment
2. gum surgery
3. placement of new dentures
4. removal of a tooth
5. temporomandibular joint treatment
6. placement of a crown
7. placement of a dental implant
8. a flap operation
9. a gingivectomy
10. periodontal treatment
11. placement of a bridge
12. extraction of an impacted third molar

Ⅲ. Substitute the following expressions in the example sentence.

It may be a bit uncomfortable, especially for the first day or two.
⟨painful⟩
It may be a bit painful, especially for the first day or two.

1. difficult
2. hard
3. inflamed
4. sore

〈歯周外科〉
患者には、歯周外科の後何をするべきか適切な指示を与えるべきである。

1. 歯科治療
2. 歯ぐきの手術
3. 新しい義歯の装着
4. 歯の除去
5. 顎関節治療
6. クラウンの装着
7. インプラント埋入
8. 歯肉剥離掻爬術
9. 歯肉切除術
10. 歯周治療
11. ブリッジの装着
12. 埋伏第三大臼歯の抜歯

Ⅲ．例文の下線部を次の語句に置き換えなさい。

特に最初の1日か2日は、ちょっと不快感があるかもしれません。
〈痛い〉
特に最初の1日か2日は、ちょっと痛いかもしれません。

1. 難しい
2. 難しい
3. 炎症がある
4. 痛い

5. stiff
6. numb
7. sensitive
8. swollen
9. rough
10. loose
11. tight
12. red

Ⅳ. Substitute the following expressions in the example dialogue.

- How about eating? May I eat today?
- You may eat if you like.
⟨sleeping⟩
- How about sleeping? May I sleep today?
- You may sleep if you like.

1. smoking
2. eating hard foods
3. taking a sauna bath
4. jogging
5. brushing my teeth
6. flossing my teeth
7. going to a movie
8. playing golf
9. playing tennis
10. drinking beer

5. 堅い
6. しびれ
7. 過敏である
8. 腫れる
9. （手触りが）荒い
10. 緩い
11. きつい
12. 赤い

Ⅳ．例にあげた対話の下線部を次の語句に置き換えなさい。

－食事はどうでしょう。今日は、食べてもよろしいですか。
－食べたいなら食べてもけっこうです。
〈眠ること〉
－眠ることはどうでしょう。今日は、眠ってもよろしいですか。
－眠りたいなら眠ってもけっこうです。

1. たばこを吸うこと
2. 堅い食べ物を食べること
3. サウナ風呂に入ること
4. ジョギングすること
5. 歯を磨くこと
6. 歯をフロスすること
7. 映画に行くこと
8. ゴルフをすること
9. テニスをすること
10. ビールを飲むこと

11. eating curry rice

12. working

Ⅴ. Substitute the following expressions in the example dialogue.

- Should I take the antibiotics even if it doesn't hurt?
- Yes. You must take the antibiotics even if there is no discomfort.

⟨stay in bed⟩

- Should I stay in bed even if it doesn't hurt?
- Yes. You must stay in bed even if there is no discomfort.

1. rest all day
2. take medicine
3. return to the clinic
4. see a doctor
5. consult a dentist
6. go to the hospital
7. change the bandage
8. brush my teeth
9. have an X-ray taken
10. wash the wound
11. keep the cut clean
12. stay at home

11．カレーライスを食べること
12．働くこと

Ⅴ．例にあげた対話の下線部を次の語句に置き換えなさい。

－痛くなくても、抗生物質をのんだ方がいいのですか。
－ええ。不快感がなくても、抗生物質はのまなければいけません。

〈ベッドで寝ている〉
－痛くなくても、ベッドで寝ていた方がいいのですか。
－ええ。不快感がなくても、ベッドで寝ていなければいけません。

1．１日中休む
2．薬をのむ
3．診療所にもう一度来る
4．医者に行く
5．歯科医に相談する
6．病院に行く
7．包帯を取り換える
8．歯を磨く
9．エックス線写真を撮ってもらう
10．傷を洗う
11．切り傷をきれいにしておく
12．家にいる

Chapter 7

The need for restoring the primary dentition

It's Only a Baby Tooth.

Most patients today realize the value of maintaining the primary dentition until natural exfoliation. However, occasionally a parent may request that you extract a primary tooth rather than fill it. The dentist explains the reasons for restoring primary teeth in this dialogue.

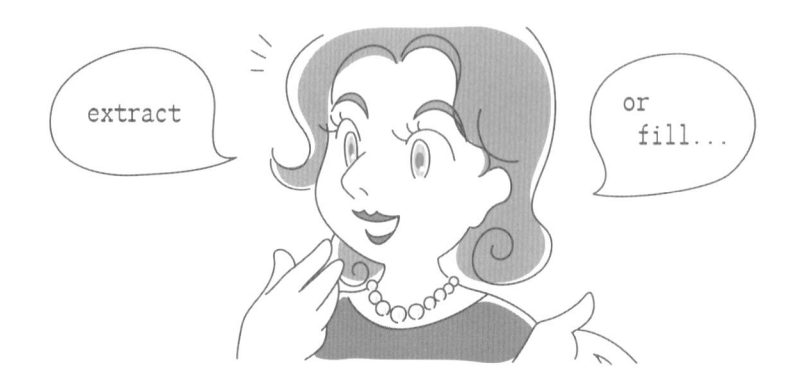

extract

or fill...

第 7 章

乳歯修復の必要性

ただの乳歯でしょう

　今では、患者の多くは、自然脱落まで乳歯を維持することの重要性を認識している。しかし、時折、乳歯を充填するより抜いてほしいと言う患者もいる。この対話では、歯科医が、乳歯を修復する理由を説明する。

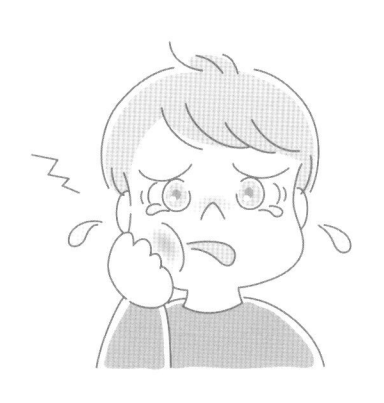

Situation: Jimmy Johnson, a six-year-old Danish boy, has a toothache in the lower left second primary molar. His mother is talking with the dentist.

Dentist: Jimmy's back tooth needs root canal treatment and a stainless steel crown.
Mrs. Johnson: It is only a baby tooth. Why don't you just pull it? He will get a permanent tooth later anyway.
Dentist: Pulling the tooth would take care of the immediate problem, but it would create a lot of other problems later.
Mrs. Johnson: What do you mean?
Dentist: That tooth should remain in his mouth about another six years. If it is taken out now, the six-year molar behind it, which is a permanent tooth, would move forward into the space.
Mrs. Johnson: What's wrong with that?
Dentist: Then the permanent teeth that come in later will not have enough space. The teeth will be crooked on that side and Jimmy will need braces when he is a teenager.
Mrs. Johnson: I don't want that. I heard that braces are expensive.
Dentist: The treatment is not cheap and the social health insurance system does not pay for it.
Mrs. Johnson: I guess it would be better to fill the tooth rather than pull it.

場面：6歳のデンマーク人坊や、ジミー・ジョンソンは、下顎左側第二乳臼歯に歯痛がある。彼の母親と歯科医が話している。

歯科医：ジミーの奥歯は、根管治療とステンレスクラウンが必要ですね。

ジョンソン夫人：ただの乳歯でしょう。抜いていただけませんか。どっちみち、後で永久歯が生えてきますし。

歯科医：現在の問題は、歯を抜けば解決しますが、後で、もっといろいろ問題が出てくることになりますよ。

ジョンソン夫人：どういうことでしょうか。

歯科医：その歯は、後6年ほど口の中にあった方がいいのです。もし今の時点で抜いてしまうと、その後ろの6歳臼歯が、これは永久歯なんですが、抜けた場所の方へと前へ動いてきます。

ジョンソン夫人：どうしてそれがいけないんでしょうか。

歯科医：すると、後で生えてくる永久歯のスペースが十分ではなくなるんです。そちら側の歯が曲がって生えてくるので、ティーンエージャーになった時、ジミーは矯正装置が必要になるでしょう。

ジョンソン夫人：それは困りますわ。矯正装置は高いと聞きましたから。

歯科医：その治療は安くはありませんし、保険もききませんよ。

ジョンソン夫人：それじゃあ、歯を抜くよりも、詰める方が良さそうですね。

Exercises

Ⅰ. Substitute the following expressions in the example sentence.

Most patients today realize the value of <u>maintaining the primary dentition</u>.
〈keeping their teeth〉
Most patients today realize the value of <u>keeping their teeth</u>.

1. regular checkups
2. preventive treatment
3. fluoride
4. brushing their teeth
5. good dentistry
6. a good hygienist
7. periodontal treatment
8. radiographs
9. floss
10. root planing
11. nutrition
12. endodontics

Ⅱ. Substitute the following expressions in the example sentence.

The dentist explained the reasons for <u>restoring the primary tooth</u>.
〈root canal treatment〉

練習問題

Ⅰ．例文の下線部を次の語句に置き換えなさい。

今では、患者の多くは、乳歯を維持することの重要性を認識している。
〈歯を保存すること〉
今では、患者の多くは、歯を保存することの重要性を認識している。

1. 定期検診
2. 予防的処置
3. フッ化物
4. 歯を磨くこと
5. 良い歯科医療
6. 良い衛生士
7. 歯周治療
8. エックス線写真
9. フロス
10. ルートプレーニング
11. 栄養
12. 歯内療法

Ⅱ．例文の下線部を次の語句に置き換えなさい。

歯科医が、乳歯を修復する理由を説明した。

〈根管治療〉

The dentist explained the reasons for root canal treatment.

1. brushing
2. periodontal surgery
3. the rubber dam
4. a flap operation
5. the plaque disclosing solution
6. gingivoplasty
7. anesthetic
8. orthodontic treatment
9. braces
10. scaling
11. bitewing X-rays
12. fluoridation

Ⅲ. Substitute the following expressions in the example sentence.

Jimmy will need braces.
⟨extensive treatment⟩
Jimmy will need extensive treatment.

1. a cleaning
2. the braces removed
3. a new retainer
4. a crown
5. a plastic filling
6. a composite resin restoration

歯科医が、根管治療の理由を説明した。

1. ブラッシング
2. 歯周外科
3. ラバーダム
4. 歯肉剥離搔爬術
5. プラーク染色剤
6. 歯肉整形術
7. 麻酔
8. 矯正治療
9. 矯正装置
10. スケーリング
11. 咬翼法エックス線写真
12. フロリデーション

Ⅲ．例文の下線部を次の語句に置き換えなさい。

ジミーは矯正装置が必要になるでしょう。
〈広範囲にわたる治療〉
ジミーは広範囲にわたる治療が必要になるでしょう。

1. クリーニング
2. 矯正装置をとり外すこと
3. 新しいリテーナー
4. クラウン
5. プラスチック充填
6. コンポジットレジン修復

7. a better tooth brush
8. a root canal
9. a silver filling
10. an amalgam restoration
11. orthodontic treatment
12. brushing instructions

Ⅳ. Substitute the following expressions in the example sentence.

I heard that braces are expensive.
⟨dental treatment⟩
I heard that dental treatment is expensive.

1. a porcelain fused-to-metal crown
2. a gold filling
3. orthodontic treatment
4. braces (are)
5. crowns (are)
6. medicine
7. root canal treatment
8. dentures (are)
9. bridges (are)
10. antibiotic medication
11. sealants (are)
12. gum surgery

7. もっと良い歯ブラシ
8. 根管治療
9. 銀の充填
10. アマルガム修復
11. 矯正治療
12. 歯ブラシ指導

Ⅳ．例文の下線部を次の語句に置き換えなさい。

<u>矯正装置</u>は高いと聞きました。
〈歯科治療〉
<u>歯科治療</u>は高いと聞きました。

1. 金属焼付ポーセレンクラウン
2. 金の充填物
3. 矯正
4. 矯正装置
5. クラウン
6. 医学
7. 根管治療
8. 義歯
9. ブリッジ
10. 抗生物質
11. シーラント
12. 歯ぐきの手術

Ⅴ. Substitute the following expressions in the example sentence.

I guess it would be better to <u>fill</u> the tooth rather than pull it.
⟨restore⟩
I guess it would be better to <u>restore</u> the tooth rather than pull it.

1. save
2. treat
3. do root canal treatment on
4. place a crown on
5. do gum surgery on
6. place a filling in
7. do a restoration in
8. do orthodontic treatment on
9. maintain
10. place a stainless steel crown on
11. place an amalgam filling in
12. place an inlay in

Ⅴ．例文の下線部を次の語句に置き換えなさい。

それじゃあ、歯を抜くより詰める方が良さそうですね。
〈修復する〉
それじゃあ、歯を抜くより修復する方が良さそうですね。

 1. 抜けないようにする
 2. 治療する
 3. 根管治療する
 4. クラウンを装着する
 5. 歯ぐきの手術をする
 6. 充填する
 7. 修復をする
 8. 矯正治療をする
 9. 維持する
10. ステンレスクラウンを装着する
11. アマルガム充填を入れる
12. インレーを入れる

Chapter 8

Consultation for orthodontics

Why Does My Daughter Need Her Teeth Straightened?

Many parents do not understand the need for orthodontic treatment. The following dialogue explains orthodontics in simple terms which most people can understand. Showing case records of orthodontic treatment while talking with the parent can be very effective.

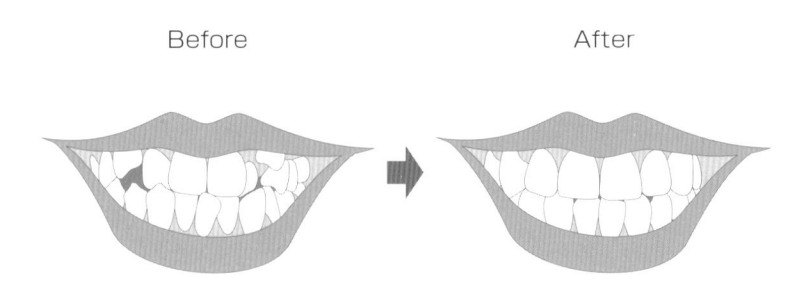

Before　　　　　　After

第 8 章

矯正治療の相談

なぜ私の娘は歯並びをなおす必要があるんですか

　矯正の必要性を理解しない親が多い。以下の対話は、ほとんどの人にわかる簡単な言葉で、矯正を説明したものである。患者と話す時には、矯正の症例記録を見せるのも非常に効果的だろう。

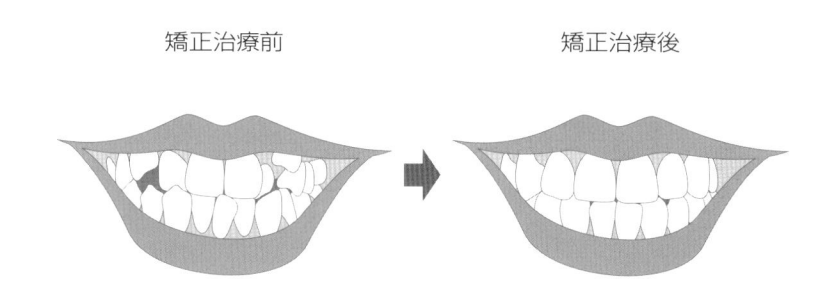

矯正治療前　　　　　　　　矯正治療後

Situation: Mary Brandt, a thirteen-year-old German girl, has class II malocclusion with bad crowding. Her father does not understand why orthodontics is necessary. In order to explain the reason for orthodontic treatment, the dentist is showing him pictures of patients which he has treated.

Mr. Brandt: Mary's teeth look OK to me. Why does she need braces?
  Dentist: There are two major problems. First, the teeth are very crowded.
Mr. Brandt: What is wrong with that? She has no trouble eating.

  Dentist: Basically, the teeth are too big for the size of the jaw. Crowded teeth are difficult to brush. This can cause problems with cavities and create gum disease later in life.
Mr. Brandt: Is that the only problem?
  Dentist: The second major problem is that the relationship of the upper teeth to the lowers is incorrect. The upper teeth are two far forward and the lower front teeth are actually touching the gums behind the upper teeth.
Mr. Brandt: What does that mean?
  Dentist: This could cause problems in the jaw joint later in life. Also, there could be pain in the roof of the mouth where the lower teeth are touching the upper gums.
Mr. Brandt: That doesn't sound very good.

場面：13歳のドイツ人少女、メリー・ブラントは叢生をともなう不正咬合（クラスⅡ）があるが、父親はなぜ矯正が必要か理解できない。矯正治療をする理由を説明するために、歯科医は、以前に処置した患者の写真を見せている。

ブラント氏：メリーの歯は私には問題ないように見えますが、なぜ矯正装置がいるのですか。
歯科医：大きな問題が2つあります。まず、歯がとても混みあっていますね。
ブラント氏：それがどうしていけないのですか。別に食べるのにさしつかえありませんけれど。
歯科医：根本的に、歯が顎の大きさに対して大きすぎます。歯が混みあっていると、磨きにくいのです。これは、後になって、むし歯の問題や、歯ぐきの病気を引き起こす可能性があります。
ブラント氏：問題はそれだけですか。
歯科医：第2の大きな問題は、上の歯と下の歯の関係が正しくないことです。上の歯が前へ出すぎているし、下の前歯は、実際に上の歯の歯ぐきにあたっています。

ブラント氏：それはどういうことですか。
歯科医：これは、後になって、顎関節に問題を起こす可能性があります。また、下の歯が上の歯にあたっている所の口蓋に痛みが出ることもあります。

ブラント氏：あまり良くなさそうですね。

Dentist: Here are some pictures taken before and after treatment of a case similar to Mary's.

Mr. Brandt: That's amazing. The teeth sure look a lot better.

Dentist: Not only is the appearance improved, but also the function is better.

Mr. Brandt: I suppose that Mary should have braces.

歯科医：ここにメリーさんに似たケースの治療前と治療後の写真が何枚かあります。
ブラント氏：すごいですね。歯が本当に見違えるようですね。
歯科医：外見が改善されるだけでなく、機能も良くなりますよ。
ブラント氏：メリーは矯正装置をつけた方が良さそうですね。

Exercises

Ⅰ. Substitute the following expressions in the example sentence.

Many parents do not understand the need for <u>orthodontics</u>.
⟨braces⟩
Many parents do not understand the need for <u>braces</u>.

1. preventive dentistry
2. restoring primary teeth
3. taking care of their children's teeth
4. regular visits to the dentist
5. early treatment
6. flossing
7. treating small cavities
8. prophylactic antibiotics
9. fluoride treatments
10. pit and fissure sealants
11. orthodontic treatment
12. disclosing solution

Ⅱ. Substitute the following expressions in the example sentence.

What is wrong with <u>crowded teeth</u>?
⟨window crowns⟩
What is wrong with <u>window crowns</u>?

練習問題

Ⅰ．例文の下線部を次の語句に置き換えなさい。

矯正の必要性を理解しない親が多い。
〈矯正装置〉
矯正装置の必要性を理解しない親が多い。

1. 予防歯学
2. 乳歯を修復すること
3. 子どもたちの歯の手入れをすること
4. 歯科医を定期的に訪れること
5. 早期治療
6. フロスすること
7. 小さなむし歯を治療すること
8. 予防のための抗生物質
9. フッ化物の応用
10. 小窩裂溝シーラント
11. 矯正治療
12. プラーク染色剤

Ⅱ．例文の下線部を次の語句に置き換えなさい。

叢生歯がどうしていけないのですか。
〈額縁冠〉
額縁冠がどうしていけないのですか。

1. my teeth
2. composite resins in posterior teeth
3. rotated teeth
4. fluoride
5. bad occlusion
6. cuspal interferences
7. extruded teeth
8. tilted teeth
9. supernumerary teeth
10. bleeding gums
11. maxillary protrusion
12. premature contacts

Ⅲ. Substitute the following expressions in the example sentence.

This could cause problems in the jaw joint later in life.
⟨periodontium⟩
This could cause problems in the periodontium later in life.

1. gums
2. teeth
3. dentition
4. permanent dentition
5. adult teeth
6. occlusion
7. alignment of the teeth
8. temporomandibular joint

1. 私の歯
2. 後方歯のコンポジットレジン
3. 回転歯
4. フッ化物
5. 不正咬合
6. 咬頭干渉
7. 挺出歯
8. 傾斜歯
9. 過剰歯
10. 出血する歯ぐき
11. 上顎突出
12. 早期接触

Ⅲ．例文の下線部を次の語句に置き換えなさい。

後になって、顎関節に問題を起こす可能性があります。
〈歯周組織〉
後になって、歯周組織に問題を起こす可能性があります。

1. 歯ぐき
2. 歯
3. 歯列
4. 永久歯
5. 大人の歯
6. 咬合
7. 歯並び
8. 顎関節

9. appearance of the teeth
10. apical region
11. periodontal tissues
12. furcation

Ⅳ. Substitute the following expressions in the example sentence.

That's amazing. The <u>teeth</u> sure look a lot better.
〈smile〉
That's amazing. The <u>smile</u> sure looks a lot better.

1. central incisor
2. front teeth
3. gums
4. periodontium
5. alignment of the teeth
6. occlusion
7. restoration
8. mouth
9. patient
10. permanent teeth
11. patient's smile
12. child's teeth

9．歯の外見
10．根尖部
11．歯周組織
12．分岐

Ⅳ．例文の下線部を次の語句に置き換えなさい。

すごいですね。歯が本当に見違えるようですね。
〈笑顔〉
すごいですね。笑顔が本当に見違えるようですね。

 1．中切歯
 2．前歯
 3．歯ぐき
 4．歯周組織
 5．歯並び
 6．咬合
 7．修復物
 8．口
 9．患者
10．永久歯
11．患者の笑顔
12．子どもの歯

Ⅴ. Substitute the following expressions in the example sentence.

I suppose that she should <u>have the work done</u>.
⟨have the teeth fixed⟩
I suppose that she should <u>have the teeth fixed</u>.

1. have the crowding corrected
2. see a dentist
3. have her teeth cleaned
4. get the tooth restored
5. have a new bridge made after treatment
6. begin orthodontic treatment
7. have her teeth straightened
8. have her teeth banded and wired for braces
9. take better care of her teeth
10. use a retainer after treatment
11. use a toothbrush and floss, even with braces
12. take care of her oral health

Ⅴ．例文の下線部を次の語句に置き換えなさい。

彼女はその治療をしてもらった方が良さそうですね。
〈歯をなおしてもらう〉
彼女は歯をなおしてもらった方が良さそうですね。

1. 叢生歯をなおしてもらう
2. 歯医者に行く
3. 歯をクリーニングしてもらう
4. 歯を修復してもらう
5. 治療後、新しいブリッジを作ってもらう
6. 矯正治療をはじめてもらう
7. 矯正してもらう
8. 矯正装置をつけるために、バンドでまいてワイヤーをつける
9. 彼女の歯をもっと大事にする
10. 治療後、リテーナーを使う
11. 矯正装置をしていても歯ブラシとフロスを使う
12. 口腔の健康を大事にする

Chapter 9

An explanation of teeth whitening

I Want to Have My Teeth Whitened.

Teeth whitening is becoming very popular in the United States and Europe. Before doing any kind of esthetic dentistry it is important that the patient be given a detailed explanation of how the treatment will be done and what results can be expected.

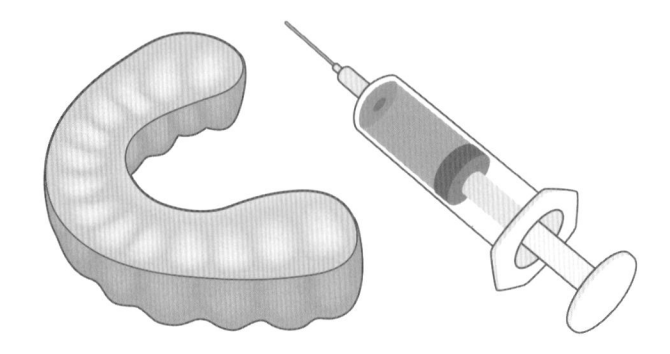

第 9 章

ホワイトニングの説明

歯を白くしたいです

　アメリカやヨーロッパではホワイトニングが非常にポピュラーになっている。審美歯科治療を行う場合は必ず、治療がどのように行われるか、またどのような結果が得られるのかについて患者に詳細な説明をすることが重要である。

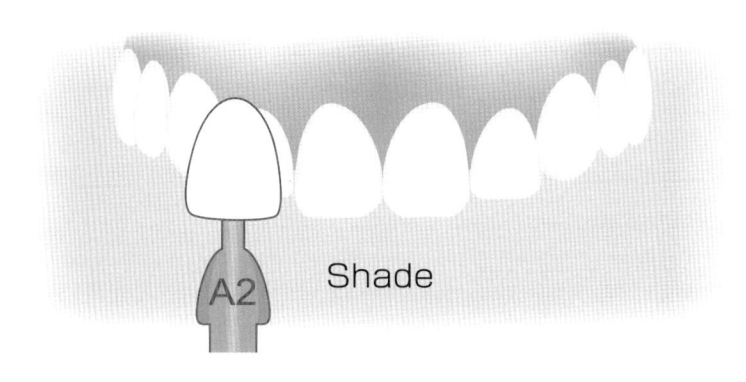

Situation: Ms. Flannigan, who is from Ireland, is asking the dentist what she can do to make her teeth whiter.

Ms. Flannigan: I don't like my teeth. They are too yellow. Can you make them whiter?
Dentist: Certainly. First let's take a look at your teeth. This is a shade guide.
Ms. Flannigan: What is that?
Dentist: The shade guide allows me to compare your teeth to standard shades of teeth. With this information, I can predict what results you might expect from whitening.
Ms. Flannigan: My teeth are too yellow.
Dentist: The basic shade of your teeth now is about A3. It is a normal shade for an adult.
Ms. Flannigan: But all my friends are having their teeth bleached, and they look so nice.
Dentist: By doing the whitening, you could certainly get the shade to A2 and maybe even A1.

Ms. Flannigan: That would be wonderful. Then I would look like a CNN announcer.
Dentist: I don't know that the teeth would get that white, but they would certainly look much better.

Ms. Flannigan: How is the whitening done?
Dentist: There are two methods. One is done in the office and one is done at home.
Ms. Flannigan: Could you tell me about them?

場面：アイルランド人のフラニゲンさんは、自分の歯をもっと白くするにはどうしたらいいか歯科医に尋ねている。

フラニゲン：自分の歯が気に入りません。あまりに黄色すぎるからです。白くしてもらうことはできますか？
歯科医：もちろん。まず、ちょっと歯を見てみましょう。これはシェードガイドというものです。
フラニゲン：それは何ですか？
歯科医：このシェードガイドで、あなたの歯の色と標準的な歯の色を比較することができます。これから得られる情報をもとに、ホワイトニングした後、あなたの歯がどのようになるか予測することができるのです。
フラニゲン：私の歯は黄色すぎます。
歯科医：あなたの歯の基本的なシェードは、だいたいA-3ですね。成人の標準的なシェードですよ。
フラニゲン：でも、私の友だちはみんなブリーチしてもらっているので、歯がとてもきれいです。
歯科医：ホワイトニングすれば、あなたの歯もA-2のシェードから、さらにはA-1のシェードにすることもできると思いますよ。
フラニゲン：すてきですね。そうなれば、私もCNNのアナウンサーのように見えますね。
歯科医：あなたの歯があれほど白くなるかどうかはわかりませんが、確かに、今よりきれいに見えるようになるでしょう。
フラニゲン：ホワイトニングって、どうするのですか？
歯科医：2通りの方法があります。1つは歯科医院で行うもの、もう1つは家で行うものです。
フラニゲン：それぞれの方法について教えていただけますか？

Dentist: Certainly. For the home whitening method, I make small transparent plastic trays that fit on your teeth. You put a small amount of bleach in the trays every evening and wear them while you sleep.

Ms. Flannigan: How many times do I have to do that?

Dentist: About twenty times are needed to complete the treatment.

Ms. Flannigan: That is too much trouble. Is there an easier way?

Dentist: Most people prefer the in-office whitening.

Ms. Flannigan: How does that work?

Dentist: It takes two appointments of about one hour each.

Ms. Flannigan: What do you do?

Dentist: I put a strong solution of bleach on the teeth and expose them to this light. The treatment is repeated two weeks later.

Ms. Flannigan: Is that all?

Dentist: Yes. But first you must have your teeth cleaned by the hygienist.

Ms. Flannigan: I want to start right away.

歯科医：わかりました。ホームホワイトニングをする場合は、あなたの歯にフィットする透明なプラスチックの小さなトレイを作ります。あなたは毎晩そのトレイにブリーチ剤を少量入れて、寝ている間装着します。

フラニゲン：何回ぐらいする必要があるのですか？
歯科医：治療が終わるまでには20回ぐらいは必要になります。

フラニゲン：たいへんすぎますね。もっと簡単な方法はありますか？
歯科医：たいていの人はオフィスホワイトニングを選びます。
フラニゲン：それはどうやるのですか？
歯科医：この場合、だいたい１時間ほどのアポイントが２回必要になります。
フラニゲン：どんなことをするのですか？
歯科医：歯に強力なブリーチ剤を塗布してこの光にあてます。この治療を２週間後にもう一度繰り返します。

フラニゲン：それだけですか？
歯科医：そうです。でも、最初に歯科衛生士に歯をクリーニングしてもらわなければいけません。
フラニゲン：今すぐ始めてください。

Exercises

I. Substitute the following expressions in the example sentence.

Tooth whitening is becoming very popular.
〈implants〉
Implants are becoming very popular.

1. composite resin restorations
2. esthetic dentistry
3. fluoride toothpaste
4. porcelain crowns
5. painless dentistry
6. international dental conferences
7. adhesive resins
8. my dental office
9. in-office bleaching
10. periodontal treatment
11. porcelain inlays
12. cosmetic dentistry

II. Substitute the following expressions in the example sentence.

All my friends are having their teeth bleached, and their teeth look so nice.
〈dental treatment〉
All my friends are having dental treatment, and their teeth look

練習問題

Ⅰ．例文の下線部を次の語句に置き換えなさい。

ホワイトニングは非常にポピュラーになっています。
〈インプラント〉
インプラントは非常にポピュラーになっています。

1. コンポジットレジン修復
2. 審美歯科
3. フッ化物配合歯磨剤
4. ポーセレンクラウン
5. 無痛（歯科）治療
6. 国際歯科会議
7. 接着性レジン
8. 私の歯科医院
9. オフィスブリーチング
10. 歯周治療
11. ポーセレンインレー
12. 美容歯科

Ⅱ．例文の下線部を次の語句に置き換えなさい。

私の友だちはみんなブリーチしてもらっているので、歯がとてもきれいです。
〈歯科治療〉
私の友だちはみんな歯科治療をしてもらっているので、歯がとて

so nice.

1. porcelain crowns
2. esthetic dentistry
3. porcelain veneers
4. cosmetic dental treatment
5. dental makeovers
6. cosmetic surgery
7. implants
8. their teeth cleaned
9. treatment here
10. teeth whitening
11. their teeth whitened
12. their amalgam fillings removed

Ⅲ. Substitute the following expressions in the example sentence.

It takes <u>two</u> appointments of about <u>one hour</u> each.
〈three/thirty minutes〉
It takes <u>three</u> appointments of about <u>thirty minutes</u> each.

1. four/forty-five minutes
2. three/one hour
3. two/two hours
4. four/fifteen minutes
5. two/five minutes
6. five/one or two hours

もきれいです。

1. ポーセレンクラウン
2. 審美歯科治療
3. ポーセレンベニア
4. 美容歯科治療
5. 口腔全体の審美歯科治療
6. 美容外科
7. インプラント
8. 歯のクリーニング
9. ここで治療
10. ホワイトニング
11. 歯を白く
12. アマルガム充填物を除去

Ⅲ．例文の下線部を次の語句に置き換えなさい。

この場合、だいたい<u>1時間</u>ほどのアポイントが<u>2回</u>必要になります。
〈3回/30分〉
この場合、だいたい<u>30分</u>ほどのアポイントが<u>3回</u>必要になります。

1. 4回/45分
2. 3回/1時間
3. 2回/2時間
4. 4回/15分
5. 2回/5分
6. 5回/1〜2時間

7. three or four/one hour
8. a few/twenty minutes
9. one or two/forty-five minutes
10. seven/one hour
11. one dozen/thirty minutes
12. three/ten minutes

Ⅳ. Substitute the following expressions in the example sentence.

First you <u>must</u> have your teeth cleaned by the hygienist.

⟨should⟩
First you <u>should</u> have your teeth cleaned by the hygienist.

1. might
2. had best
3. ought to
4. will
5. will likely
6. will most likely
7. are going to
8. should always
9. had better
10. will need to
11. might need to
12. would like to

7. 3〜4回/1時間
 8. 数回/20分
 9. 1〜2回/45分
10. 7回/1時間
11. 12回/30分
12. 3回/10分

Ⅳ．例文の下線部を次の語句に置き換えなさい。

最初に歯科衛生士に歯をクリーニングしてもらわ<u>なければ</u>いけません。
〈〜べき〉
最初に歯科衛生士に歯をクリーニングしてもらう<u>べき</u>です。

 1. （もらって）ください
 2. （もらうのが）一番よい
 3. （もらう）べきです
 4. （もらう）ことになります
 5. （もらう）ことになるでしょう
 6. （もらう）可能性が高いでしょう
 7. （もらう）ことになりそうです
 8. いつも（もらう）べきです
 9. （もらった）方がいいでしょう
10. （もらう）必要があるでしょう
11. （もらう）必要があるかもしれません
12. （もらい）たい

V. Substitute the following expressions in the example dialogue.

－What should I do about my teeth?
－First let's <u>take a look at the teeth</u>.
⟨do a cleaning⟩
－What should I do about my teeth?
－First let's <u>do a cleaning</u>.

1. do anterior composite resin restorations
2. remove the stain
3. do a dental examination
4. brush the teeth
5. do a fluoride treatment
6. examine the problem
7. remove the amalgam
8. treat the pain
9. take radiographs
10. remove the calculus
11. see the dental hygienist
12. remove the plaque

Ⅴ．例にあげた対話の下線部を次の語句に置き換えなさい。

－自分の歯に何をすればいいのですか？
－まず、ちょっと歯を診てみましょう。
〈クリーニングする〉
－自分の歯に何をすればいいのですか？
－まず、クリーニングしましょう。

 1．前歯にコンポジットレジン修復をする
 2．ステインを除去する
 3．歯科検診をする
 4．歯を磨く
 5．フッ化物を塗布する
 6．問題を検討する
 7．アマルガムを除去する
 8．痛みをなおす
 9．エックス線写真を撮る
10．歯石を除去する
11．歯科衛生士と会う
12．プラークを除去する

Chapter 10

Advising a patient about implant treatment

What Can I Do about that Missing Tooth?

Implants have become a reliable and predictable treatment for restoration of function and esthetics where there are missing teeth. Because most patients do not understand implant treatment, it is often helpful to draw a picture of the teeth showing what will be done.

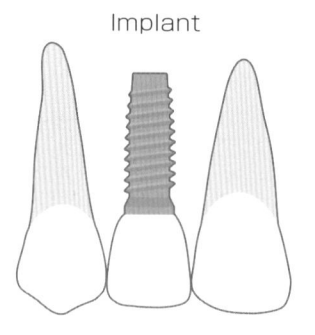

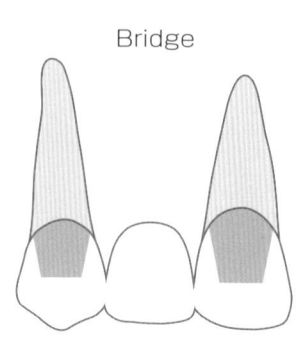

Implant   Bridge

第 10 章

インプラント治療についてのアドバイス

歯を失った場合、どうすればいいのですか

　インプラントは、失った歯の機能や審美性の修復を目的とした信頼のおける予知性の高い治療となった。しかし、多くの人はインプラントをよく理解していない。そこでどのような治療がされるのか、歯の絵を描くと役に立つことが多いようだ。

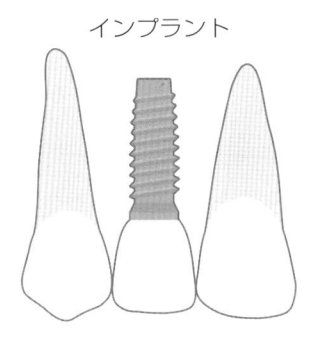

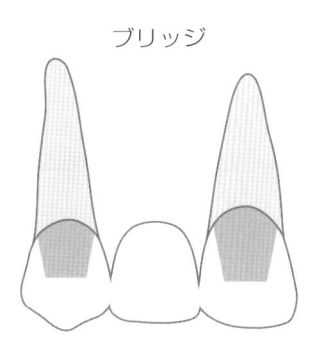

インプラント　　　　ブリッジ

Situation: Ms. Ivanova is an Estonian flight attendant for a European airline. She is based in Tokyo, and wants to have implant treatment for a missing maxillary anterior tooth that was lost in a traffic accident.

Ms. Ivanova: I have this removable plastic front tooth and it is not comfortable. Can you recommend something more permanent?
Dentist: The best treatment for this case is probably a dental implant.
Ms. Ivanova: What is that?
Dentist: A dental implant is a small titanium post that is placed in the bone. Please look at this drawing.
Ms. Ivanova: Now I can understand. But does it hurt?
Dentist: No, not at all. It only takes a few minutes to place the implant, and it is done with local anesthetic.
Ms. Ivanova: Does it hurt after the anesthetic wears off?
Dentist: It might be a little uncomfortable for a day or two afterwards, but you can take pain pills for that.
Ms. Ivanova: That's not so bad.
Dentist: An artificial porcelain tooth is later placed on top of the implant.
Ms. Ivanova: How long will the implant last?
Dentist: The titanium implant may last a lifetime. However, the crown on the implant may need to be replaced a few times.
Ms. Ivanova: How about a bridge. Wouldn't that be easier?

場面：イバノバーさんはヨーロッパの航空会社に勤めるエストニア人のフライトアテンダントです。彼女は東京を本拠地としており、交通事故で失った上顎前歯をインプラントで治療したいと思っています。

イバノバー：前歯に入れ歯が入ってるいのですが、具合よくありません。もう少し耐久性のあるものはありませんか？

歯科医：この場合、たぶんインプラント治療がもっとも適した治療でしょう。

イバノバー：それはどんなものですか？

歯科医：歯科用のインプラントとは小さなチタン製のポストで、それを骨に植立します。この絵を見てください。

イバノバー：ええ、よく理解できました。でも、痛くないですか？

歯科医：少しも痛くありません。インプラントを植立するのには数分しかかかりませんし、局所麻酔をしますから。

イバノバー：麻酔が切れてから痛くなりませんか？

歯科医：1〜2日は少し不快感があるかもしれませんが、その場合は痛み止めの薬を飲めばいいのです。

イバノバー：悪くないですね。

歯科医：後でインプラントの上にポーセレンの人工歯を装着します。

イバノバー：インプラントはどれぐらい持ちますか？

歯科医：チタンインプラントは生涯もつでしょう。しかし、インプラントの上のクラウンは数回取り替える必要があるかもしれません。

イバノバー：ブリッジにするのはどうですか？　その方が簡単なのではないですか？

Dentist: I don't recommend a bridge for this case.

Ms. Ivanova: Why not?

Dentist: If you place a bridge it is necessary to cut down the two teeth on either side to attach the artificial tooth. This is unnecessary with an implant.

Ms. Ivanova: I don't want to cut down good teeth.

Dentist: I agree with you.

Ms. Ivanova: An implant seems like the best treatment.

Dentist: I also think that would be best for you.

歯科医：あなたの場合、ブリッジは勧められません。
イバノバー：どうしてですか？
歯科医：ブリッジを入れる場合、人工歯の両隣の歯を2本とも削らなければならなくなります。インプラントならその必要はありません。
イバノバー：いい歯を削りたくはないですね。
歯科医：同感です。
イバノバー：インプラントが一番いい治療のようですね。
歯科医：それが一番だと私も思います。

Exercises

I. Substitute the following expressions in the example sentence.

Implants have become a reliable and predictable treatment.
〈periodontal surgery〉
Periodontal surgery has become a reliable and predictable treatment.

1. composite resin restorations
2. gingival graft surgery
3. porcelain crowns
4. implant surgery
5. cosmetic surgery
6. fluoride applications
7. gold inlays
8. porcelain inlays
9. root canal therapy
10. endodontic surgery
11. ultrasonic scaling
12. root planing

II. Substitute the following expressions in the example sentence.

A bridge is necessary for restoration of function and esthetics.
〈inlay〉
An inlay is necessary for restoration of function and esthetics.

練習問題

Ⅰ．例文の下線部を次の語句に置き換えなさい。

インプラントは信頼のおける予知性の高い治療となりました。
〈歯周外科〉
歯周外科は信頼のおける予知性の高い治療となりました。

1. コンポジットレジン修復
2. 歯周形成術
3. ポーセレンクラウン
4. インプラント外科
5. 美容外科
6. フッ化物塗付
7. ゴールドインレー
8. ポーセレンインレー
9. 根管治療
10. 歯内外科治療
11. 超音波スケーリング
12. ルートプレーニング

Ⅱ．例文の下線部を次の語句に置き換えなさい。

機能性と審美性を回復するためにはブリッジが必要です。
〈インレー〉
機能性と審美性を回復するためにはインレーが必要です。

1. crown
2. posterior composite restoration
3. occlusal restoration
4. interproximal restoration
5. composite resin restoration
6. porcelain-fused-to-metal crown
7. anterior bridge
8. bone graft
9. implant
10. porcelain inlay
11. composite resin filling
12. porcelain crown

Ⅲ. Substitute the following expressions in the example sentence.

The best treatment for this case is probably a dental implant.
⟨extraction of the tooth⟩
The best treatment for this case is probably extraction of the tooth.

1. removal of the tooth
2. a bone graft
3. periodontal surgery
4. orthodontics
5. a porcelain bridge
6. minor tooth movement
7. antibiotics

1. クラウン
2. 臼歯部のコンポジット修復
3. 咬合面修復
4. 隣接面修復
5. コンポジットレジン修復
6. 金属焼付ポーセレン
7. 前歯部ブリッジ
8. 骨移植
9. インプラント
10. ポーセレンインレー
11. コンポジットレジン充填
12. ポーセレンクラウン

Ⅲ．例文の下線部を次の語句に置き換えなさい。

この場合、たぶんインプラント治療がもっとも適した治療でしょう。
〈抜歯〉
この場合、たぶん抜歯がもっとも適した治療でしょう。

1. 抜歯
2. 骨移植
3. 歯周外科
4. 矯正治療
5. ポーセレンブリッジ
6. MTM（部分矯正）
7. 抗生物質

8. full mouth reconstruction
9. teeth whitening
10. root planing
11. surgical orthodontics
12. endodontic surgery

Ⅳ. Substitute the following expressions in the example dialogue.

－How about a bridge. Wouldn't that be easier?

－I don't recommend a bridge for this case.
⟨an inlay⟩
－How about an inlay. Wouldn't that be easier?

－I don't recommend an inlay for this case.

1. a gold crown
2. a removable partial denture
3. orthodontics
4. endodontic surgery
5. a plastic crown
6. amalgam
7. a Maryland bridge
8. antibiotics
9. having the tooth extracted
10. an extraction
11. whitening

8. フルマウス・リコンストラクション
9. ホワイトニング
10. ルートプレーニング
11. 外科矯正治療
12. 歯内外科治療

Ⅳ．例にあげた対話の下線部を次の語句に置き換えなさい。

－<u>ブリッジ</u>にするのはどうですか？　その方が簡単なのではないですか？
－この場合、<u>ブリッジ</u>は勧められません。
〈インレー〉
－<u>インレー</u>にするのはどうですか？　その方が簡単なのではないですか？
－この場合、<u>インレー</u>は勧められません。

1. ゴールドクラウン
2. 可撤性部分床義歯
3. 矯正治療
4. 歯内外科治療
5. レジンクラウン
6. アマルガム
7. メリーランドブリッジ
8. 抗生物質
9. 抜歯すること
10. 抜歯
11. ホワイトニング

12. composite resin

V. Substitute the following expressions in the example dialogue.

- How long will the implant last?
- It will likely last a lifetime.
⟨filling/five or ten years⟩
- How long will the filling last?
- It will likely last five or ten years.

1. porcelain crown/ten or twenty years
2. composite resin/five or ten years
3. tooth/a few more years
4. gold inlay/fifteen or twenty years
5. plastic crown/three or four months
6. dental treatment/several years
7. bridge/ten years
8. denture/five years
9. old filling/a year or two
10. denture repair/a few months
11. treatment/only a few months
12. new restoration/for several decades

12．コンポジットレジン

Ⅴ．例にあげた対話の下線部を次の語句に置き換えなさい。

－<u>インプラント</u>はどれぐらい持ちますか？
－インプラントは<u>生涯</u>持ちます。
〈充填物/5〜10年〉
－<u>充填物</u>はどれぐらい持ちますか？
－充填物は<u>5〜10年</u>持ちます。

1．ポーセレンクラウン/10〜20年
2．コンポジットレジン/5〜10年
3．歯/2〜3年以上
4．ゴールドインレー/15〜20年
5．レジンクラウン/3〜4ヵ月
6．歯科治療/数年
7．ブリッジ/10年
8．義歯/5年
9．古い充填物/1〜2年
10．修理した義歯/数ヵ月
11．治療/わずか数ヵ月
12．新しい補綴物/数十年

Chapter 11

The use of foreign dental insurance

Is the Cost Covered by Insurance?

Many foreigners in Japan have dental insurance through private insurance companies in their home country. The insurance usually reimburses the patient for 50 to 70% of the cost of their dental treatment. The patient may ask you to fill out a form listing treatment and costs after the work is completed. It is best to have the patient pay you directly when the work is done. The insurance company will pay him back later.

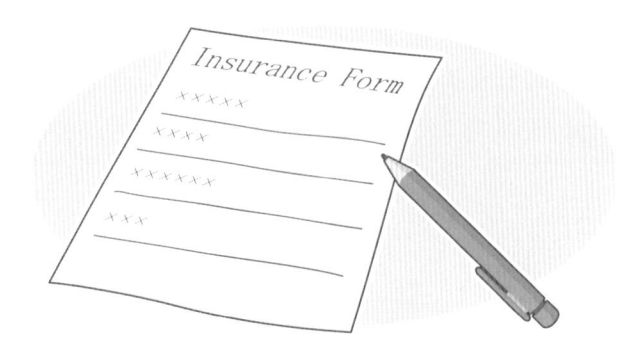

第11章

外国の歯科保険の使用

その治療費は保険がききますか

　日本にいる外国人の多くは、本国の保険会社の歯科保険を持っている。通常、その保険は、歯科治療費の50〜70％を患者に払い戻すものである。治療後、治療内容とその費用を用紙に書き入れるように、患者から頼まれるかもしれない。治療後、患者に直接支払ってもらうのが一番良い。保険会社は、後で、患者に払い戻しをする。

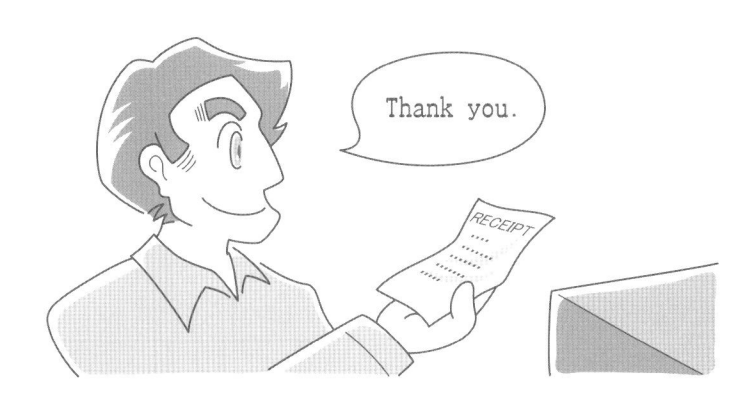

Situation: Mr. Butler who is employed by an international pharmaceutical company, is asking about using his American dental insurance at the clinic.

Mr. Butler: Can I use this insurance at this office?
Dentist: Certainly. We often treat patients here who have that type of insurance.
Mr. Butler: Does the insurance company pay you directly?
Dentist: No. It is necessary for you to pay for the treatment when it is done. My secretary will give you a receipt and fill out the form for the insurance company.

Mr. Butler: How much money will they give me back?
Dentist: I do not know. Each company is different. Usually they will reimburse you about 50 to 70% of the cost of the treatment.
Mr. Butler: That's not so bad. Let's get started with the examination.

場面：国際的製薬会社に勤めているバトラー氏が、診療所でアメリカの歯科保険使用について尋ねている。

バトラー：ここではこの保険が使えますか。
歯科医：もちろんです。ここでは、よくそういった型の保険をお持ちの患者さんを治療しています。
バトラー：保険会社が直接先生に支払うのですか。
歯科医：いいえ。治療の代金は、完了した時に患者さんに払っていただかなければなりません。事務の者が領収書をあなたにさしあげて、保険会社に出す用紙に書き入れます。
バトラー：会社はどのくらい支払ってくれるんでしょうか。
歯科医：私にはわかりかねます。会社によって違いますから。普通は、治療費の50〜70%を払い戻してくれますが。

バトラー：悪くはないですね。じゃあ診察をはじめましょうか。

Exercises

Ⅰ. Substitute the following expressions in the example sentence.

The patient may ask you to fill out a form.
⟨clean his teeth⟩
The patient may ask you to clean his teeth.

1. fill out an insurance form
2. list the treatment
3. fill in the blanks on the form
4. write your address on the form
5. restore his teeth
6. do a routine examination
7. write a letter for the insurance company
8. give him a receipt
9. give him a discount
10. examine his children's teeth
11. take X-rays
12. avoid taking X-rays

Ⅱ. Substitute the following expressions in the example sentence.

It is best to have the patient pay you directly.
⟨pay in yen⟩
It is best to have the patient pay in yen.

練習問題

Ⅰ．例文の下線部を次の語句に置き換えなさい。

<u>用紙に書き入れる</u>ように、患者に頼まれるかもしれない。
〈歯をきれいにする〉
<u>歯をきれいにする</u>ように、患者に頼まれるかもしれない。

1. 保険用紙に書き入れる
2. 治療内容を書く
3. 用紙の空欄に書き入れる
4. 用紙に住所を書く
5. 歯を修復する
6. 定期検診をする
7. 保険会社に手紙を書く
8. 彼に領収書を渡す
9. 値引きをする
10. 彼の子どもの歯を診察する
11. エックス線写真を撮る
12. エックス線写真を撮らない

Ⅱ．例文の下線部を次の語句に置き換えなさい。

患者に<u>直接支払って</u>もらうのが一番良い。
〈円で支払う〉
患者に<u>円で支払って</u>もらうのが一番良い

1. brush his teeth three times each day
2. floss every day
3. use a synthetic bristle toothbrush
4. wear the dentures only during the day
5. clean his dentures every day
6. return every six months for a regular checkup
7. rest after an extraction
8. eat soft foods
9. use an interproximal brush
10. rest after periodontal surgery
11. take medication
12. consult a specialist

Ⅲ. Substitute the following expressions in the example sentence.

It is necessary for you to pay for the <u>treatment</u> when it is done. 〈crowns〉

It is necessary for you to pay for the <u>crowns</u> when they are done.

1. bridge
2. periodontal treatment
3. porcelain crown
4. cleaning
5. surgery
6. amalgam restoration
7. composite resin restorations

1. 毎日3回歯を磨く
2. 毎日フロスする
3. 合成繊維の歯ブラシを使う
4. 日中だけ義歯をはめる
5. 毎日義歯をきれいにする
6. 6ヵ月ごとに定期検診にやってくる
7. 抜歯の後で休む
8. 軟らかい食物を食べる
9. 歯間ブラシを使う
10. 歯周外科の後休む
11. 薬をのむ
12. 専門家に相談する

Ⅲ．例文の下線部を次の語句に置き換えなさい。

治療の代金は、完了した時に払っていただかなければなりません。
〈クラウン〉
クラウンの代金は、完了した時に払っていただかなければなりません。

1. ブリッジ
2. 歯周治療
3. ポーセレンクラウン
4. クリーニング
5. 手術
6. アマルガム修復
7. コンポジットレジン修復

8. prosthodontic treatment
9. root canal treatment
10. non-insurance treatment
11. restorations
12. gold crown

Ⅳ. Substitute the following expressions in the example sentence.

My secretary will give you a receipt.
⟨a call⟩
My secretary will give you a call.

1. a telephone call
2. an appointment
3. my Fax number
4. the completed insurance form
5. a letter of recommendation
6. an appointment card
7. a receipt for the treatment
8. a bill
9. a card to fill out
10. my name card
11. the office telephone number
12. the name of an orthodontist

8. 補綴治療
9. 根管治療
10. 自由診療の治療
11. 修復
12. 金冠

Ⅳ．例文の下線部を次の語句に置き換えなさい。

事務の者が領収書をあなたにさしあげます。
〈電話〉
事務の者が電話をあなたにさしあげます。

1. 電話
2. 予約
3. ファックス番号
4. 記入済みの保険用紙
5. 推薦状
6. 予約カード
7. その治療の領収書
8. 請求書
9. 書き入れるカード
10. 私の名刺
11. 診療所の電話番号
12. 矯正歯科医の名前

Ⅴ. Substitute the following expressions in the example sentence.

Let's get started with the <u>examination</u>.
⟨treatment⟩
Let's get started with the <u>treatment</u>.

1. surgery
2. periodontal surgery
3. endodontic treatment
4. preparation of the tooth
5. brushing instructions
6. occlusal adjustment
7. gum surgery
8. oral surgery
9. removal of plaque
10. cleaning
11. oral prophylaxis
12. root planing

Ⅴ．例文の下線部を次の語句に置き換えなさい。

診察をはじめましょうか。
〈治療〉
治療をはじめましょうか。

1. 手術
2. 歯周外科
3. 歯内療法
4. 歯の形成
5. ブラッシング指導
6. 咬合調整
7. 歯ぐきの手術
8. 口腔外科手術
9. プラークの除去
10. クリーニング
11. 口腔清掃
12. ルートプレーニング

Chapter 12

Explaining the social insurance system to a foreigner

Can I Use My Social Insurance Card Here?

Recently there are many foreigners who desire treatment under the Japanese social insurance system. Before starting treatment, it is important to explain the cost they must pay. Also, they should realize that the social insurance system does not pay for porcelain crowns or gold restorations.

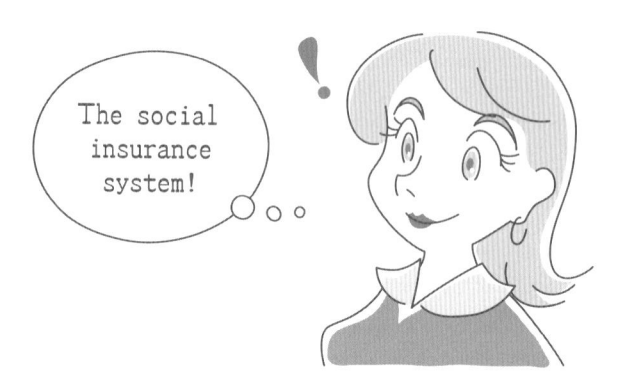

The social insurance system!

第 12 章

外国人に社会保険制度を説明する

ここでは、社会健康保険証が使えますか

　最近、日本の健康保険で治療を希望する外国人も多い。治療を始める前に、患者が負担しなければならない費用について説明することが大切である。社会保険は、ポーセレンクラウンや貴金属修復物にはきかないということを、患者が認識しておくべきである。

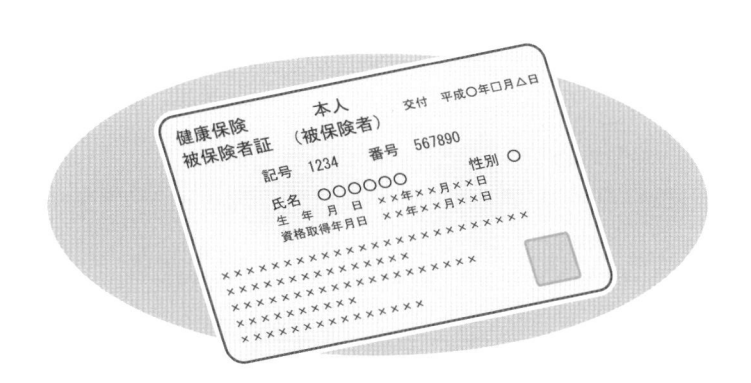

Situation: Mrs. Starky, an English teacher from Australia, would like to have all of her dental work done using her social insurance card. The dentist is explaining the treatment plan and the costs.

Mrs. Starky: Can you do all of this treatment under the social insurance system?

Dentist: Under this system you are required to pay about 10% of the cost of the basic treatment※. Since the fees specified by the government are very low, you will be paying only a few thousand yen for the examination, cleaning, X-rays, and fillings.

Mrs. Starky: That is very cheap.

Dentist: However, the insurance will not pay for the bridge you need on the front teeth.

Mrs. Starky: Why not? I pay a lot of money each month for this insurance.

Dentist: The insurance will not pay for porcelain. If you want the front teeth to look natural, they must be made of porcelain.

Mrs. Starky: What will the insurance pay for then?

Dentist: You have three choices, none of which is very satisfying.

Mrs. Starky: What are my choices?

Dentist: The front teeth could be restored with a metal bridge.

Mrs. Starky: I don't want that. It would look terrible.

Dentist: Otherwise, I could put in a small removable denture

※患者負担率は時代により異なります。

場面：オーストラリア人の英語教師、スターキーさんは、すべての治療を保険を使ってしてもらうことを希望している。歯科医は治療計画と費用を説明する。

スターキー：治療はすべて健康保険でできますか。

歯科医：この制度では、基本的治療の約10％を負担していただく必要があります。政府が定めた料金は非常に低いので、支払いは、診察、クリーニング、エックス線写真、充填で2〜3千円だけですみます。

スターキー：それはたいへん安いですね。
歯科医：でも、あなたの場合、前歯に必要なブリッジには保険はききません。
スターキー：なぜですか。この保険に、毎月たくさんお金を支払っていますのに……。
歯科医：保険はポーセレンにはきかないんですよ。もし、前歯が自然に見える方が良いのなら、ポーセレンで作らないといけません。
スターキー：それじゃあ、保険がきくのはどんなものですか。
歯科医：3つの中から選べますが、どれもあまり満足のいくものじゃあないですよ。
スターキー：どのようなものですか。
歯科医：前歯は、メタルブリッジで修復することもできます。

スターキー：そんなのはいりませんわ。すごく不格好ですもの。
歯科医：そうでなければ、プラスチックベースの、小さな取

with a plastic base. It would not look very good, but it would fill the gap.

Mrs. Starky: I don't want anything like that. What is the third choice?

Dentist: You can do nothing — just leave the gap unrestored.

Mrs. Starky: That is out of the question. I guess I will have to pay for the porcelain bridge.

りはずしのきく義歯を入れることもできます。それもあんまり格好良くありませんが、隙間はうめることになりますからね。

スターキー：そういうのもごめんですわ。3番目のは何ですか。

歯科医：何もしないこと。つまり歯の抜けた後をそのままにしておくことです。

スターキー：それは論外ですわ。ポーセレンブリッジのお金を払うより他ないみたいですね。

Exercises

Ⅰ. Substitute the following expressions in the example sentence.

You should realize that the social insurance system does not pay for porcelain crowns.
⟨metal base dentures⟩
You should realize that the social insurance system does not pay for metal base dentures.

1. everything
2. regular checkups with X-rays
3. gold crowns
4. gold inlays
5. orthodontic treatment
6. regular cleaning
7. periodic oral prophylaxis
8. 100% of the cost of treatment
9. unnecessary treatment
10. toothbrushes
11. dental floss
12. braces

Ⅱ. Substitute the following expressions in the example sentence.

She would like to have the treatment done soon.
⟨medicine⟩

練習問題

Ⅰ．例文の下線部を次の語句に置き換えなさい。

社会保険は、<u>ポーセレンクラウン</u>にはきかないということを認識しておくべきである。
〈メタルベースデンチャー〉
社会保険は、<u>メタルベースデンチャー</u>にはきかないということを認識しておくべきである。

1. すべてのもの
2. エックス線写真付の定期検診
3. 金冠
4. ゴールドインレー
5. 矯正治療
6. 定期的クリーニング
7. 定期的口腔清掃
8. 治療費の100％
9. 不必要な治療
10. 歯ブラシ
11. デンタルフロス
12. 矯正装置

Ⅱ．例文の下線部を次の語句に置き換えなさい。

彼女は、<u>すぐに治療をしてもらう</u>ことを希望している。
〈薬〉

She would like to have medicine.

1. insurance treatment
2. private treatment
3. free treatment
4. an insurance card
5. a new bridge
6. a cleaning
7. an extraction
8. the suture removed
9. the crown replaced
10. an examination
11. the inflammation treated
12. the denture relined

Ⅲ. Substitute the following expressions in the example sentence.

I pay a lot of money each month for this insurance.
〈dental treatment〉
I pay a lot of money each month for dental treatment.

1. toothbrushes
2. interproximal brushes
3. dental insurance
4. medical insurance
5. dentistry
6. medicine

彼女は薬を希望している。

1. 保険治療
2. 自費治療
3. 無料の治療
4. 保険証
5. 新しいブリッジ
6. クリーニング
7. 抜歯
8. 抜糸
9. クラウンを取りかえて
10. 診察
11. 炎症を治療して
12. 義歯を裏装して

Ⅲ．例文の下線部を次の語句に置き換えなさい。

私はこの保険に、毎月たくさんお金を支払っています。
〈歯科治療〉
私は歯科治療に、毎月たくさんお金を支払っています。

1. 歯ブラシ
2. 歯間ブラシ
3. 歯科保険
4. 医療保険
5. 歯科医療
6. 薬

7. insurance
8. health care
9. my dental care
10. maintaining my oral health
11. dental floss
12. dental supplies

Ⅳ. Substitute the following expressions in the example sentence.

The front teeth could be restored with <u>a metal bridge</u>.
⟨composite resin⟩
The front teeth could be restored with <u>composite resin</u>.

1. gold
2. a partial denture
3. amalgam
4. crowns
5. porcelain fused-to-metal crowns
6. porcelain
7. resin jacket crowns
8. new crowns
9. silicate
10. porcelain laminate
11. inlays
12. post crowns

7. 保険
8. 健康維持
9. デンタルケア
10. 口腔健康管理
11. デンタルフロス
12. 歯科器材

Ⅳ．例文の下線部を次の語句に置き換えなさい。

前歯は、メタルブリッジで修復することもできます。
〈コンポジットレジン〉
前歯は、コンポジットレジンで修復することもできます。

1. 金
2. 部分義歯
3. アマルガム
4. クラウン
5. 金属焼付ポーセレンクラウン
6. ポーセレン
7. レジン・ジャケットクラウン
8. 新しいクラウン
9. 珪酸セメント
10. ポーセレンラミネート
11. インレー
12. ポストクラウン

Ⅴ. Substitute the following expressions in the example dialogue.

- Would you like a metal bridge?
- That is out of the question.

⟨to lose your teeth⟩

- Would you like to lose your teeth?
- That is out of the question.

1. to have insurance treatment
2. to extract the tooth
3. dentures
4. gum surgery
5. silver fillings
6. to have the tooth extracted
7. to neglect your teeth
8. to have braces
9. to get gum disease
10. to use floss every day
11. to have a toothache
12. to stop smoking

Ⅴ．例にあげた対話の下線部を次の語句に置き換えなさい。

－メタルブリッジにしたいですか。
－それは論外です。
〈歯を失うこと〉
－歯を失いたいですか。
－それは論外です。

 1. 保険治療をすること
 2. 歯を抜くこと
 3. 義歯
 4. 歯ぐきの手術
 5. 銀の充填物
 6. 歯を抜くこと
 7. 歯のケアを怠る
 8. 矯正装置をすること
 9. 歯ぐきの病気になること
10. 毎日フロスを使うこと
11. 歯痛になること
12. 禁煙すること

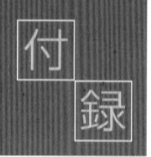

患者とのコミュニケーションで役立つ最重要用語100語

以下は、患者とのコミュニケーションに役立つ最重要用語100語を、アルファベット順に並べたものである。これらは特に歯科用語を知らない人にもわかる言葉である。

A

ache	痛む、痛み
adjust	合わせる、調整する
adjustment	調整
amalgam	アマルガム
amalgam filling	アマルガム充填物
anesthetic	麻酔薬
antibiotics	抗生物質
appointment	予約、アポイント、約束

B

baby tooth	乳歯
back tooth	奥歯
bacteria	細菌
bite	噛む、咬合
bitewing	咬翼
bleed	出血する
bleeding	出血
braces	矯正装置
bridge	架工義歯

C

calculus	歯石
canine	犬歯
cavity	むし歯、窩洞
cement	セメント
checkup	（歯科）検診
chew	噛む
cleaning	（歯の）清掃
clinic	診療所
consultation	診察、相談
contacts	（歯の）接触
crowding	叢生

crown	歯冠、クラウン			
cusp	咬頭	gap	隙間	
		gums	歯ぐき	

D

decay	むし歯		**H**	
dental	歯科の、歯の	heal	治癒する	
denture	義歯	hurt	痛む	
diagnosis	診断	hygienist	衛生士	
discomfort	不快			
disease	疾患		**I**	
		impacted	埋伏している	
	E	impression	印象	
effective	有効な、効果がある	infected	感染した	
enamel	エナメル質	infection	感染	
erupt	萌出する	inflamed	炎症性の	
examination	予診、診査	inflammation	炎症	
examine	診察する	inflammatory	炎症性の	
extract	抜く	injection	注射	
extraction	抜去			
			J	
	F	jaw	顎	
fee	報酬、料金			
fill	充填する		**L**	
filling	充填（物）	lower tooth	下顎の歯	
floss	フロス、糸			
flossing	フロッシング		**M**	
fluoride	フッ化物	medication	薬	
fracture	破折、骨折	molar	臼歯	
front tooth	前歯			
function	機能			

0167

付録

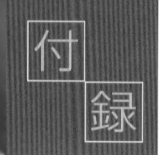

N
nerve	神経
nutrition	栄養

O
operation	手術、処置
orthodontist	矯正歯科医

P
patient	患者
permanent tooth	永久歯
plaque	プラーク
prevent	予防する
preventive	予防の

R
receptionist	受付係
relieve	軽減する
retainer	保定装置、リテーナー
root canal	根管

S
sealants	シーラント
sensitive	敏感な
social insurance	社会保険
specialist	専門医
stain	有色性沈着物、着色
straighten teeth	歯列矯正
surgery	外科学、外科
swelling	腫脹
symptom	病状、症状

T
tablet	錠剤
temporary	暫間の
tissue	組織
toothache	歯痛
treatment	治療、処置

U
uncomfortable	不愉快な
upper tooth	上顎の歯

W
wisdom tooth	智歯

X
X-ray	エックス線

クインテッセンス出版の書籍・雑誌は，歯学書専用通販サイト『歯学書.COM』にてご購入いただけます．

PCからのアクセスは…
歯学書　検索

携帯電話からのアクセスは…
QRコードからモバイルサイトへ

QUINTESSENCE PUBLISHING 日本

改訂版　クインテッセンス歯科英会話シリーズ
PART1 英語で患者と話そう！

1989年5月10日　第1版第1刷発行
2007年8月10日　第2版第1刷発行
2020年1月15日　第2版第3刷発行

著　　　者　Thomas R. Ward（トーマス　アール　ウォード）

発　行　人　北峯康充

発　行　所　クインテッセンス出版株式会社
　　　　　　東京都文京区本郷3丁目2番6号　〒113-0033
　　　　　　クイントハウスビル　電話　(03)5842-2270(代表)
　　　　　　　　　　　　　　　　　　　(03)5842-2272(営業部)
　　　　　　　　　　　　　　　　　　　(03)5842-2279(編集部)
　　　　　　web page address　https://www.quint-j.co.jp/

印刷・製本　サン美術印刷株式会社

©2007　クインテッセンス出版株式会社　　　　禁無断転載・複写
Printed in Japan　　　　　　　　　　　　　　落丁本・乱丁本はお取り替えします
ISBN978-4-87417-967-3　C3047　　　　　　　定価はカバーに表示してあります